STYLE SISTERS

yellow kite

HELPING YOU
LIVE AN *organised*
& *stylish* LIFE

STYLE SISTERS

Gemma Lilly and Charlotte Reddington

contents

introduction

A HELLO FROM US

A big hello and warm welcome to our debut book! We're Gemma and Charlotte, and together we're the Style Sisters, an organising and styling duo specialising in fashion, styling and interiors. We started Style Sisters together back in 2018 and since then it's been the most incredible journey to get to where we are today. We always envisioned Style Sisters as a lifestyle brand covering every aspect of what you need to live a stylish and practical life. Style Sisters was built on our love of organising, fashion and interiors, and a passion for helping people – and this is still the case today. We get such a buzz working on our clients' homes and sharing those feelings of calm, satisfaction and joy that they get from their totally refreshed space.

This book is for anyone who wants to transform the way they feel in their home and about their home for the better, for those of you who want more space in your life, visually and emotionally, who want to let go of all the 'stuff' that's getting in the way. This is our toolkit for working your way out of the chaos – for those of you who, like our clients, need some some Style Sisters magic to get them out of a clutter and style rut. Whatever your budget, these are accessible tools for detoxing, streamlining and adding back some sparkle. By following our process, you're one step closer to becoming the most organised person you know.

You're going to get a snapshot of how we work, who we are and what we believe in, and we're going to have a lot of fun along the way. We will show you that bit by bit, you can do the most seemingly overwhelming tasks and make the changes that will make life that little bit easier to navigate.

HOW IT ALL BEGAN

We were both born in 1987 with the same middle name and both of our children's dads share the same surname, so people often joke that we are the same person and, to be honest, we can't really argue with that!

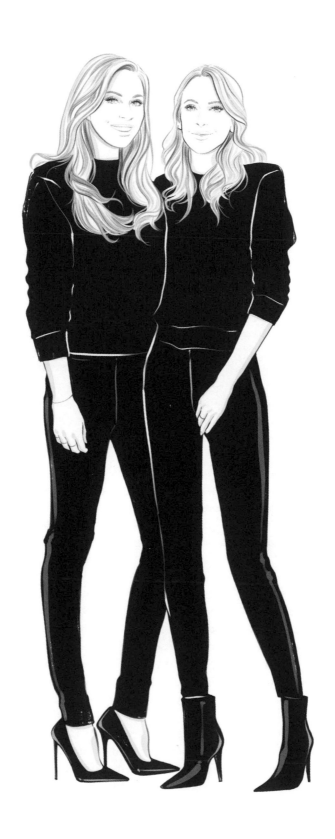

We are similar in so many ways but most importantly in our style, values and work ethic. We both have big dreams but started on totally different paths before Style Sisters was born. We became friends at sixth-form college, both taking the same subjects, proving that, from the very start, our interests were in sync. Gemma started her career in fashion and Charlotte in interiors, and although fashion and interiors are closely linked, it hadn't occurred to either of us that we could merge the two and do something amazing together. We both only completed the first year of sixth form, quickly realising it wasn't for us. Charlotte went off to start a successful career in PR and Gemma went to fashion college.

It wasn't until a few years later that we discovered via Facebook that we were pregnant at the same time and were only seven weeks apart. We were the first in our friendship group to have kids and it was nice to know we had each other. This definitely set us on the path to becoming best friends, with our boys growing up to be best friends too!

At this point, Charlotte was doing interiors for local clients and Gemma had her own fashion boutique and was freelance styling for brands. We would push, support and encourage each other on our respective paths but both felt we had so much more to give.

OUR DREAMS

It was over dinner and cocktails one night that we had the light-bulb moment to merge what we were doing. We were feeling a little frustrated with the direction our careers were going in. We knew we could make it bigger and better and have a lot more fun with it. It was in that moment that Style Sisters was born!

We always knew we wanted a business name that was short, catchy and versatile and that had the room to grow. With each of us bringing experience from lots of different avenues, we didn't want to pigeonhole ourselves. We wrote down lots of words that represented us and what we are about and played around with putting all of the words together. As soon as we saw 'Style Sisters' we just knew that was the name for us. We wanted to be like the sisters who come in to help you with all your organising and styling needs – we loved that 'sisters' felt comforting and friendly and not intimidating, which was important to us given the services we were offering. Having people come into your personal space can feel daunting, overwhelming and even embarrassing, and we never want anyone to feel ashamed for asking for help. We always want to put everyone at ease and reassure them – we have literally seen it all and nothing could scare us or make us judge a client. We always joke, 'the messier the better' and this couldn't be more true – we actually get a bit disappointed if things are quite tidy when we turn up, we love to get stuck into a project!

THE POWER OF SOCIAL MEDIA

Once we had our business name, the next day, after getting in from the school run, we set up our Style Sisters Instagram account. Within an hour a friend sent us a screenshot of a *Love Island* contestant asking for someone to help her organise her wardrobe. We never thought that messaging to offer our services would pay off, especially since our Instagram had next to no followers or posts of our work, but we didn't have anything to lose and by that afternoon we had our very first (celebrity) client! This definitely set the pace from the word go. From then on, the business grew quickly through word of mouth. We always say it was meant to be, as for the first time in a long time it didn't feel like we were forcing something to be great, it just was.

It was incredible to see the business grow so rapidly and to reach the kind of clientele we had always dreamed of, from the likes of Vicky Pattison and Ferne McCann to Rochelle Humes and Amanda Holden. Word was spreading fast due to the power of social media and our before and after Instagram pictures, which gave our followers never-seen-before, behind-the-scenes access to celebrity homes, coupled with their honest reviews. Hitting our first major milestone of 10k followers in May 2018 when the business was only two months old was huge. It felt really special to us both after all the hard work getting Style Sisters off the ground.

Although this growth appears as though it happened overnight, we spent years feeling lost and frustrated and had tried out various businesses which didn't work out and, truthfully, we can now see why. They weren't meant to be and although at the time we couldn't see it, it was a blessing in disguise. The businesses we tried, including a clothing website, beauty treatments, styling and interiors, were just a snapshot of what we enjoy doing as a whole – and doing one of these things at a time just wasn't fulfilling. Style Sisters ticks all the boxes for us. It allows us to be creative in so many areas, from styling our own photoshoots to coming up with the creative concepts for the imagery and even making our own props! We love to turn our hands to anything and give it a go. We enjoy taking a space and making it the best it can be, styling it to look amazing in the process and we are such people-pleasers, which can be both a blessing and a curse!

AN AMAZING JOURNEY

We knew straight away that we had a business that would work, and we both felt energised and excited about our new baby, from appearing on ITV's *This Morning* to regularly featuring in national newspapers and magazines. Everything was flowing, and we really feel it's because Style Sisters comes from a place of passion and love. You can always tell when someone is doing what they do because they love it and not just for the money, and this is the case for us. We have never been ruled by money and have always stayed true to ourselves and the business. We've turned down ads, sponsorships and collabs that we didn't feel were right for the business and our followers, and we will only ever work with another brand that we genuinely believe in and use ourselves. It doesn't sit with us to be fake and false, and although money is hard to turn down when it's offered, we know it's better for the business in the long run and for the vision that we have for Style Sisters.

Within a few months of setting up the business, we were approached by lots of managers offering to represent us. We signed with one but after a few months it became apparent we weren't on the same page and it felt like the business was slowing down. So, it was exciting to meet our current manager, Lauren, when the business was a year old. We naturally clicked with her and knew she had the same values and vision for Style Sisters as us. We couldn't be more grateful to have someone so like-minded to work alongside.

Since we started the business, we have spent every day completely obsessed with our brand and mission – we are the first person each other speaks to in the morning and the last person every night, even after a 12-hour working day together! Everything is run and orchestrated by us, apart from a few talented people who we work with from time to time, from photographers to make-up artists and carpenters. We are lucky to have such an amazing, close-knit, hard-working team to support us. When we leave a client's home, they often tell us how relieved they feel and how we have changed their lives. We treat every single person's home as if it is our own. We're total perfectionists and we don't leave until everything is exactly how it should be. Even when the client is ecstatic, we often message each when we get home, wondering whether we could have done something differently. We truly believe that this is why we get so many repeat clients, as we give so much time, energy and love to everything we do. After spending so much time at our clients' homes, we quickly build friendships with them, which is one of the things we love about our job. We frequently find ourselves getting emotional with clients because we fully immerse ourselves and care about curating a home that functions smoothly and makes them happy when they are in it. Something we should all have in this fast-paced world packed with pressure and endless to-do lists.

We get so many supportive messages from our clients when we hit certain milestones and it's lovely to have this support from people who have been with us on our journey from the start. We have shared fun, laughter and even tears with our clients, from Amanda Holden being the hostess with the mostess and bringing us wine to keep us going through late-night girly chats during her wardrobe detox, to Lisa Snowdon cooking us a delicious lunch and Rochelle Humes trusting us to style her baby brand shoot.

WHAT WE CAN DO TO HELP YOU

Style Sisters is our way to help people make their homes the best they can be. Our secret weapon is knowing how to make a space better, and we want to teach you how to do the same. It's important to have a home and wardrobe that reflects you, your taste and your style, which is not only aesthetically pleasing but, most importantly, functional too. Knowing everything has a home will completely change your mentality. Cutting clutter from your life is a huge weight off your shoulders and letting go of anything you no longer need makes space for better, brighter things to enter your life.

We hope you guys are ready to become addicted to our Style Sisters way! You might not think it will happen to you, none of our victims, sorry clients, do, but once you start the process, you won't want to stop. We've worked with such a vast array of clients to adapt and organise their homes, whether it's because they've had a change in lifestyle due to a new career or because they've welcomed a child and their home doesn't fit this new stage in their lives. We've had clients who are so busy that the clutter has got on top of them and they just don't know where to start. We've seen first-hand the transformative power that a calm and clear space can have when someone is going through a difficult time, when they've lost any motivation to start and it's all just too much… With this book, we want to equip you with the same advice we give our clients, so you too can feel the best version of yourself.

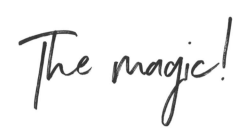

The magic!

THE MAGICAL BENEFITS OF ORGANISING AND DECLUTTERING, AND THE TRANSFORMATIVE POWER OF SIMPLE, ACHIEVABLE TASKS IN THE HOME.

In 2020, due to the pandemic, we all spent more time at home than ever before and the way that we use our spaces expanded massively... focusing on simple, achievable tasks became essential for so many of us have who have struggled in these uncertain times whilst juggling work, childcare and the added layer of health worries. But even in a 'normal' world that's super fast-paced, our routines get chaotic and it's easy to get overwhelmed mentally. Through our tips, tricks and practical advice, we want to put the power back in your hands. We want the Style Sisters Process to be to be your magic wand.

These handy solutions are exactly the same ones we use to overhaul over clients' homes and lives. By following our guidance, you'll tick off daily wins, you'll regain control and you'll stop thinking about all that stuff you can't do, instead learning to celebrate what you can do; everyday tasks that lead to better clarity and a clearer, positive outlook when everything else feels cloudy and hard. We're here to make the magic happen, and we will be there every single step of the way, telling you, YES YOU CAN.

If you commit to the Style Sisters way as a lifestyle choice, you'll of course reap the visual benefits, but the mental benefits are wonderful too – more happiness, more productivity, more time to spend doing the things you love. All in all, it will be easier to navigate your day and everything will function that little bit more smoothly, with less stress and more of the good stuff.

We have had clients who didn't think they would get much satisfaction out of an organise, but then find that it gives them and their space a new lease of life. They see the amazing benefits that decluttering brings. There's a certain indescribable feeling that everyone experiences once a space has gone from

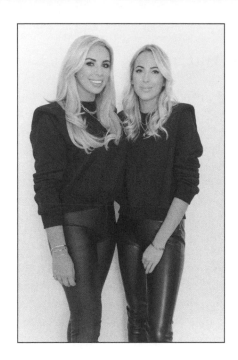

chaos to calm – the energy physically lifts a room and is infectious, addictive and rewarding.

Being organised allows your daily routine to flow, and gives you more brain space for the things that truly matter. Removing clutter gives you a push to face life in the present and future, rather than hanging on to things from the past. We take no greater satisfaction than leaving a home knowing our work has had a positive impact and we want to lead you through your home, room by room, to make it as functional and beautiful as it can be and become a place where you can spend time building good memories and associations from the moment you enter.

If you're struggling with motivation, turn your attention to the doable things first, those areas in sight that are most accessible and, in time, bit by bit, your confidence to tackle the lot will get there! Start slow – that drawer or cupboard, or finally getting rid of that item that triggers bad memories and makes you feel bad about all the to-dos you still haven't managed. Remember, this is a process, especially if you have let things get on top of you for a long while. Getting started is better than not starting at all.

Let's do this together! We promise you'll never look back.

HOW TO USE THIS BOOK

The first part of this book details everything you need to get going and covers all the need-to-know Style Sisters basics including our must-have kit to detox and style your space. We'll show you how to work out where to start and share our magic steps that you can apply to any space to transform it into a stylish, ordered haven. You'll find that by trusting in our simple step-by-step process, you'll have every corner covered. Don't think about overhauling the whole house, instead break it down into individual rooms (or doable chunks) and first decide what you would love to achieve in that particular space (see pages 18–45 for more on this stress-free approach).

In the Detox & Organise section (see pages 46–187), we share our tips and tools to declutter, organise and style every space in your home. Each chapter is dedicated to a room, kicking-off with the first place you enter as you step through the door – the hallway – working through the main living areas and then to the bedroom, bathroom and kids' rooms. There's also a special section on one of our favourite areas – the wardrobe. We share our timeless advice on what to consider when purchasing items for the wardrobe and home, and offer options for all budgets. Skip to the sections that are relevant to you and your home, but do bear in mind that there might be relevant information relating to another room you have in other chapters. For example, you may not have a dining room, but a dining table in your living room, so you can get ideas and inspiration for table styling from the Dining Room chapter.

The final part looks at how to maintain and style your space after the detox. We will encourage you to identify your unique style (see page 192), give you the confidence to trust and develop this and have some fun with it, alongside sharing our best home hacks for upcycling furniture, saving money and time, making the most of items you already own and finding clever ways to maximise storage. Although we are often designing beautiful walk-in wardrobes and other glamorous projects as the business has grown, we are just as excited by seeing someone take our advice on hangers and sharing the results on Instagram. We would absolutely love to see you share your transformations, so after reading and using this book tag us on Instagram @StyleSisters #STYLESISTERS! We want this to be a super useful and practical guide to transforming your home and outlook, and to help you to feel good from the inside out in the process.

Remember, when you start your detox and organisation, playlists and snacks are essential. Let's get started!

Top 10 Detox Tracks

We have made many memories as we've listened to these songs over the years!

1. 'Wish I Didn't Miss You' – Angie Stone
2. 'Freedom' – George Michael
3. 'This Is How We Do It' – Montell Jordan
4. 'Sunshine' – Tieks
5. 'Fantasy' – Mariah Carey
6. 'Never Too Much' – Luther Vandross
7. 'Crazy Love' – MJ Cole
8. 'Something Got Me Started' – Simply Red
9. 'U Know What's Up' – Donell Jones
10. 'The Real Thing' – Lisa Stansfield

On the job and always having fun!

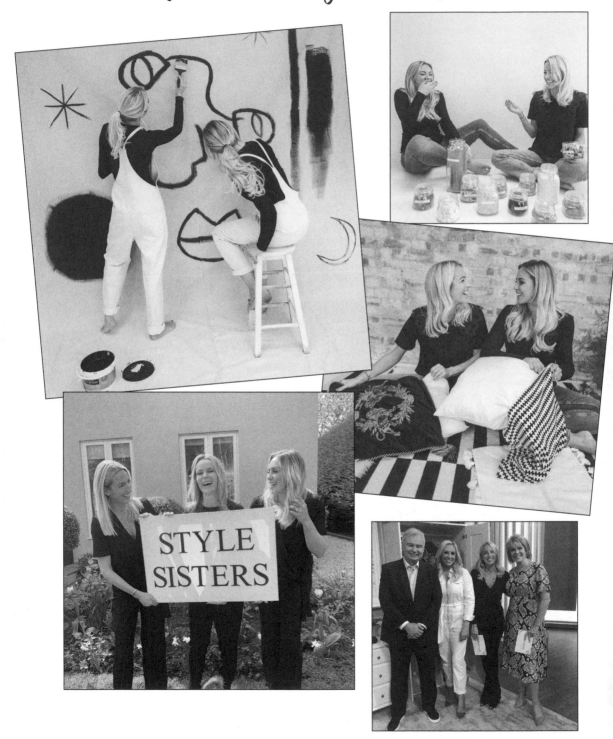

STYLE SISTERS

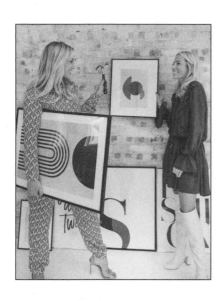
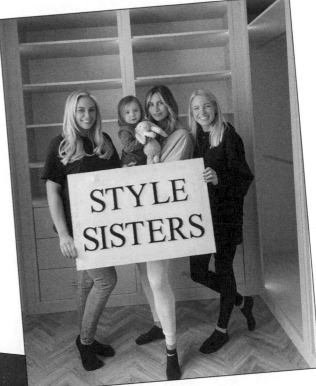

STYLE
SISTERS

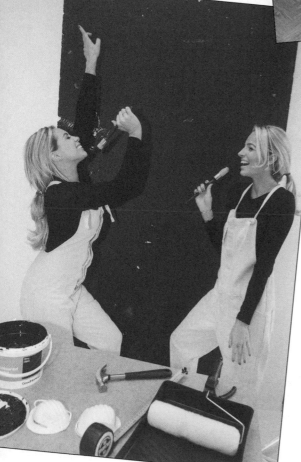
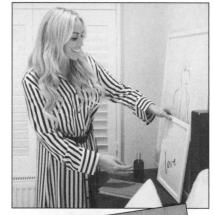
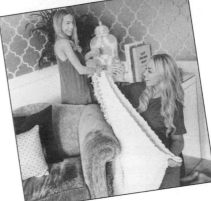

part 1
GETTING

STARTED

THE BENEFITS OF BEING ORGANISED

The benefits of getting organised, as touched on already, are abundant! We've all heard the saying 'tidy home, tidy mind', and we couldn't agree with this more.

HOME FLOW

Having a home that is not only super functional but is in sync with your lifestyle can have such a positive effect on the way your whole home flows and works together. It will also stop those family arguments about putting things away as everyone is aware of where things should go. Having a foolproof system means there's no excuse for anyone not knowing where everything lives. Providing a long-term home for every item will help everyone learn where things should go – no excuses and no more 'do you know where X is?'. This is where labels are also very helpful (more on our much-loved label machine later – see page 31)!

TIDY HOME, TIDY MIND

We love using any available space to create stylish storage around the home. Let's face it, we don't all live the minimalistic life that you see in the glossy magazines! We like to keep it real and in real life we all have too much stuff… So it's about working out which items serve a purpose and add value to your life, and then storing them in the correct place so they function as they should. Your home should contain all the things you use and love and should be organised in a way that suits your routine and needs. Having your home life flow will have such a positive effect on your mental head space when you feel like everything else is chaos. For example, your underwear drawer is something you open every day. If it's a mess and you can't find your favourite knickers (we all have a pair!), it's going to stress you out. It isn't until you've organised these clutter hot spots and detoxed everything that doesn't fit or is worn out that you realise how amazing it feels and how much it bothered you before.

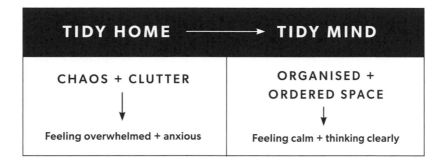

SAVE TIME

Having an organised home can save you hours and days of time. Not having to rummage around to find a particular item is a game-changer, especially when it comes to kids! Once you have children, you tend to acquire many more items, from bottles and nappy changing kits when they're babies to toys and books when they're older. Being able to find lunchboxes or a PE kit saves time and stress, especially in the morning rush of the school run! When your home is organised to suit your lifestyle, you'll be able to set up a seamless routine. If you don't have to spend time tidying or finding items, then you can focus your attention on what you need to do without getting side-tracked by clutter. You'll get back some control.

SAVE RELATIONSHIPS!

Through our Style Sisters work we have even rescued a marriage, which we know sounds crazy, but it's true! A client was at his limits with his wife's mess, which flowed from their walk-in wardrobe to the bedroom floor. Mess is a complete passion-killer, but your bedroom should also be a calm space where you can switch off and unwind. Our lives are so busy that our minds can get full of thoughts and worries really quickly, having a bedroom that is cluttered makes you feel more cluttered and self-loathing. Once we had organised and detoxed the husband and wife's space there were lots of tears of happiness. A major argument in their household had been eliminated; we all felt a sense of relief and the energy in the house completely lifted. It was an unnecessary bone of contention and a reason to nit-pick and this can foster a negative atmosphere in the home. Consider any arguments in your household that you think could be solved by introducing some organisation.

TACKLING THE TIDYING BLOCKS

The idea of organising your home so it flows may seem daunting and overwhelming, but it doesn't have to be. If we can do it, there is honestly nothing stopping you from being able to too. The toughest battle is often carving out the time, committing to the process and a willingness to let go. So, just buckle up and stick with us – we promise the results will be worth your time and energy.

Listed below are some of most the common reasons people often put off getting organised, BUT we have the solutions, so you no longer have to.

FINDING TIME

Set aside a day, or even a couple of hours, and schedule it in the diary. People often put off an urgent task because not only does the thought of it feel like climbing a mountain, but busy lives leave little time. Scheduling in your detox helps you to mentally prepare for it. It allows you to be in the right head space. To do something thoroughly and properly, you need to leave yourself enough time and be realistic. Trying to squeeze in ten minutes here and there is just going to stress you out even more and you'll end up shoving everything back where it came from!

Make a day of it, get your comfies on, put on some music (see our detox playlist on page 15) and get in the zone. You're about to clear yourself of anything that has consciously and subconsciously been weighing you down – this is an exciting opportunity!

Another option if you are really pushed for time is to tackle smaller problem areas, be it a drawer or a cupboard, these are doable chunks for your focus. The little wins will give you a taster for how good you will feel when everything is organised and will motivate you to tackle more. See page 35 for for more inspo on where to start.

KNOWING WHERE EVERYTHING SHOULD GO

Often people get confused about where items should go and so put off tackling the task at hand full stop. We can assure you that once you have specific homes for items, everything will fall into place.

The idea is that similar items are homed together and wherever an item lives needs to be somewhere relevant to where you need or use it. You wouldn't go looking for your bank statement in the bathroom cupboard. You have to think logically when placing and homing items, don't just bung them in a spare random nook because there is space in there. It needs to make sense for your home to flow in an organised and practical way.

Once you start pulling everything out in the detox phase (see pages 36–9) and you have worked out what is going to be kept, you will probably find you have fewer things to home in that room and so have room to store items from another place. The magic of pulling everything out to detox is that it's much easier to put things back. Don't be scared to change the home of something. Just because the pens have lived in the kitchen drawer since you moved in doesn't mean they have to continue to do so. Perhaps you now have a home office space, or there's an area in the living room where other stationery is being stored and they could move there too, freeing up space in the kitchen. Now the pens get to live with other stationery items happily ever after! Our detox process gives you the opportunity to see it all with fresh eyes and really think about functionality.

WHAT TO DO WITH ITEMS

We always say: 'create your categories'. This helps with the detox process as often a major block is not knowing what to do with discarded items, especially if they have sentimental value, or are something you have spent money on and don't necessarily want to just give away. Identifying key categories such as 'keep', 'give', 'sell' and 'get rid' is the perfect way to keep in check when you're mid-detox. It stops you from feeling drowned by stuff and throwing everything back where it came from. You can then have subcategories, such as a 'maybe' pile – just remember you will often be putting off the inevitable by putting things here, so try not to add too many items to this category.

Sometimes you just need to let things go and be honest with yourself. Holding on to items purely because you have spent money on them or barely used them is such a common mistake. We want everyone to realise that these unused things are taking up valuable space in your home (and mind) and they are a constant reminder of something you don't love but are just holding on to out of guilt. We always say: get honest with yourself! A common occurrence when we are working on clients' homes is them feeling guilty about parting with unused gifts. This should not be the case. They are scared that by letting these things go they seem ungrateful. This is your home and your space; you do not have to feel guilty about not wanting to home things that aren't suited to your style or taste.

We often have deep and meaningful conversations with our clients when certain items are pulled out and they have memories attached to them. This can lead to stories, laughter or tears. We had one client who had items that she had worn and purchased during her previous marriage in her wardrobe but was hesitant about getting rid of them, even though they reminded her of her old life, that broken relationship and such a different period in time. After a little pep talk from us and talking openly about it, she quickly realised that they were an unwelcome reminder, and they didn't have a place in her wardrobe or her future any more. So, she donated them to charity and felt happy that someone else would get to enjoy the clothes and have fresh experiences wearing them.

Everyone grows and changes and what may have worked well for you five years ago or even one year ago when you were in a different head space, may no longer trigger any joy... just because. You can change, you don't need permission, and giving unwanted items a new home is simply spreading the love. If you sell the item and then buy something you do love,

You do not have to feel guilty about moving on from stuff that no longer benefits you, your life, your style and your home.

Client Stories

We had one lovely client who had lost over half her body weight – going from a size 18 to a size 10. She had maintained that size for several months before we arrived to help her detox and organise her wardrobe. She was worried she was going to need her old, larger clothing in the future and wanted to keep hold of items 'just in case' and get some taken in at the seamstress as she had spent money on them. We worked alongside her throughout the day and explained that it was OK to let these clothes go. Saying goodbye to the old garments that she was no longer wearing was a positive step to saying goodbye to the old her and her worries that she would become that person again. She felt like a weight had been lifted and now only has clothes in her wardrobe that she can wear so she isn't reminded every day of the past.

this is a fruitful cycle and, if you give it away, you are sharing the gift with someone else. Knowing that items you no longer want, or need, are going to new homes where they can be loved, used or worn again will make you feel a lot better about letting them go.

If you really can't part with certain items, consider storage or memory boxes (see page 28). You can then review these at a later date when you are ready or in a better head space to move on.

'I LOVE YOU GIRLS! WHEN CAN YOU MOVE IN?!'

Rochelle Humes

'THANK YOU SO MUCH GIRLS, I CAN'T BELIEVE HOW LIFE-CHANGING THIS HAS BEEN.'

Billie Faiers

MAKE A MEMORY BOX

Memory boxes can be extremely beautiful and every client we've worked with either already had a version of one or has started one once we've been there. They are the perfect place to store a range of items that have a special meaning to you or that you're not ready to step away from, but that you don't want on display or don't have another place to store.

The type and size of memory box you will need all depends on how much you want to store in there. Always remember to work with what space you have available. Having one giant memory box but nowhere to put it is not ideal. If you are making smaller memory boxes, break them down into categories, for example cards and notes together in one, then sentimental pieces or clothes in another.

There are plenty of boxes out there that you can use for your memory box – there will always be one that suits your décor and needs. If it's going to be displayed somewhere, try to make sure it matches the theme of the room. Another lovely idea is to get creative and make your own. You can decorate a box you have around the house or you could even use an old shoe box.

There are no rights or wrongs – the goal here is to have a place to store items. It's also worth mentioning that it is very easy to get sucked in to saving every last thing! We all know that is less than practical, so be really selective and honest with yourself about why a certain item is important and what impact it would have on your long-term emotions if you were never to see it again. Does it hold an important memory? Do you enjoy looking at it? Will it make you sad if its gone? You want to keep items where the answer is 'yes' as opposed to keeping something because you are unsure, where the instinctual response is 'maybe' or it doesn't come with ease. These things don't hold the right meaning for a memory box.

REMEMBER to be mindful about what items go into your memory box as you don't want it becoming another place to store junk. Items that you may want to include:

★ *Sentimental cards, postcards or letters, including special birthday cards, Valentine's cards or thank you letters with heartfelt messages.*

★ *Pictures – these could be old photos that you don't want to display or to put in a photo album, or even children's first drawings from nursery or school.*

★ *First babygrows, booties, hats or a christening gown, a hospital wrist band from when they were born, a baby book or their first lock of hair.*

★ *Tickets or invites to memorable events and maps or other mementoes from favourite places that you've travelled to.*

★ *Clothes that don't fit, aren't your style or are slightly damaged that hold sentimental value (see page 140).*

Any item that means something to you and that you may want to look at in the future belongs in here.

We like to create a memory box for every member of the family. If you're making one for a child, you can include items from when they were a baby through various ages, including favourite toys they may have grown out of. They can then look through the box when they are older. We often get out our children's memory boxes with them now on birthdays and they enjoy looking at the things they loved and used when they were younger.

STYLE SISTERS
must-haves

These are our must-have items when it comes to organising your home. You don't have to spend hundreds of pounds on kit but investing in these bits now will be a present to your future self – thank us later! These are our go-to pieces that will make living an organised life that bit easier. Set yourself up now!

★ LABEL MACHINE

You will never have more fun than when using your trusty label machine. They will cost you around £20 but we think this is a worthwhile investment as you can use them in every single room. A little top tip – you can buy different brand labels to go in them cheaply on Amazon if purchasing in bulk. Just make sure they are compatible with your machine.

If you don't want to invest in a label machine, you can make your own handwritten ones. You can do this using sticky labels and a nice pen, or you can design labels on the computer and print them out. Your options for gorgeous labels are endless!

top tip

When labelling your children's storage, you could print out your own labels and use images such as toy cars, dolls, etc. so that the children know where to put their toys away. This way you can train them young and even make it into a fun game! Parents – 1, Kids – 0.

★ STORAGE BOXES

You can never have enough! There are lots of amazing options to suit all your needs – from decorative baskets that are patterned or plain, woven or soft fabric baskets, to paper and firmer ones. There will be a style and size that will work for you. Smaller ones are great for use in bathrooms and larger ones are perfect for places like bedrooms, living rooms and wardrobes.

Try to stick to boxes or baskets that suit the décor of your space and keep them all matching or colour-coordinated.

★ VACUUM-PACK BAGS

You can use these to store out-of-season clothes – get a variety of sizes for different storage options.

★ DRAWER DIVIDERS

Warning, after use you will keep opening drawers just to look inside and admire your hard work! There are lots of drawer divider options available; make sure you properly measure up the size before making purchases. IKEA SKUBB drawer dividers are great for deeper drawers and organising items like underwear and belts. The shallow drawer dividers from iDesign are handy for accessories, make-up and bits and bobs. If you don't want to invest in dividers, consider using empty shoe boxes or other small boxes to structure different sections within drawers.

★ SLIMLINE VELVET HANGERS

We joke that they will change your life, but we're not even joking … they really will! If you're not a fan of velvet (we've discovered some people have a phobia), you can get slimline plastic or metal hangers that you can use instead. (See page 218 for where to find these.)

★ MEMORY BOXES

Those sentimental items that you can no longer afford to give prime space to (see page 140). They can be stored away, freeing up valuable easy access space for other everyday and essential items (see page 28).

★ BIN BAGS

You need to have somewhere to put your purged items and there will definitely be rubbish. You will also need recycling bags for paper and recyclable tins/metals/plastics, depending on the recycling system in your area.

★ CLEANING PRODUCTS

We really get stuck in and get our hands dirty when we're doing a Style Sisters overhaul! We love using lovely smelling cleaning products that are non-toxic. Gloves are handy if you're using harsher, bleach-like cleaning sprays. Be mindful about using these in certain areas, especially wardrobes as you don't want to risk them causing damage or stains to clothing.

THERE ARE SO MANY BENEFITS TO LIVING AN ORGANISED LIFE – YOUR HOME WILL LOOK AMAZING AND YOU WILL FEEL AMAZING!

OUR METHOD WILL HELP YOU TRANSFORM YOUR SPACE INTO AN ORGANISED AND STYLISH HAVEN.

WHERE DO I START?

So where to begin?

Grab a notebook and pen – we want you to write a list of all the rooms in your home that you would love to organise in order of importance. Start with the room that makes most sense to you or that you feel is most in need of decluttering. Under each room, list what you want to achieve. Is it just a detox and organise or are you styling the space too? You can start from the hallway and make your way through the home (as we do in this book, see Part 2) or start from the top of the house and work down to the bottom if you have more than one floor. There really are no rules.

If, for example, you want to sort your bedroom first, then title a piece of paper 'Bedroom'. Then write down each part of the room you'd like to tackle. It might be your underwear drawer, bedside tables, make-up, etc. This way, you can start small, accomplishing as much as you have time for or can face, and you can tick off areas as you go along. These tiny wins will be encouraging and motivating, so make sure you celebrate. Much like lots of things in life, this stops you from focusing on what you haven't done. It's a positive way of approaching life's endless to-do lists and means you stop obsessing over your failure, what you're lacking or haven't still accomplished, and instead smash those micro-goals and piece together the puzzle to create a beautiful picture in the end – with time, patience and love. It doesn't matter whether you manage to organise a whole room in one day or one part of a room, making a start is all that matters. With our tips, once you have given everything a home, the process will become a breeze. It will then only ever be a space that needs maintaining, not a complete overhaul.

the PROCESS

These are our *magic* steps that you
can easily follow and apply to detoxing
and organising any room in your home.
They will help you determine what
should stay and what should go.
Whether you tackle a drawer or the
whole room, the process is exactly
the same. You can apply these to each of
the rooms as we flow through the book:

GET EVERYTHING OUT!
**We really mean it when we say get everything out! Yes, that too…
we see you!**

Don't leave any corner unturned. Whether it's your wardrobe, kitchen
cupboards or a living room sideboard, everything needs to come out to
be seen and assessed. If we're organising a kitchen, we literally empty out
every corner, but if this overwhelms you then don't worry, you can work from
cupboard to cupboard. However, this can be a bit more confusing as you
need to divide all the items into categories, so we would recommend being
brave and emptying it ALL – go on, you can do it, deep breath…

WARNING *It will get messy before it gets tidy. Just remember that this is a
process, and the end goal will be totally worth it. We always say this should
feel exciting – you're finally clearing out what is weighing you down. No more
staring at items you never use, and you will feel so zen after detoxing, we
promise you!*

2   CATEGORISE: KEEP, GIVE, SELL, GET RID

When getting everything out, place items into categories.

This is the most important step and probably the longest. Divide or label your items into four main categories: keep, give, sell, get rid. You can then create subcategories within these, i.e. for keep, you can utilise your memory box (see page 28 for more on how to make these) or put into storage. For give, there will be give to a loved one or give to charity/donate. For get rid, there will be recycle or simply, rubbish, when the item has come to the end of the road. This detox process will allow for a streamlined structure for each room. See more on how to categorise and organise under 'Contain and Label' (below).

top tip

When categorising and deciding what you want to keep and what should go, be honest with yourself. Ask yourself when the last time you used something was and how likely it is that you will use it again. If you haven't used it in the past year, it's more than likely it needs to go.

3   CLEAN

This is the perfect time to give space that you may not normally be able to get to a good wipe down and vacuum.

Once the surface or area is empty, we vacuum it to get up the main dust, then wipe over with a cloth and an antibacterial spray, which will leave it clean and smelling fresh!

4   CONTAIN AND LABEL

We kid you not, we don't think anything is more fun than using a label machine (see page 31)!

It may seem obvious, but labelling really does add value to the detox process. Labels can be used ANYWHERE in your home, from the kitchen cupboards to label what food goes on which shelf to clothing in your baby's room – once you start labelling, you won't want to stop! Not only does it help other family members acknowledge that everything has its rightful place, but it forces you to maintain all your hard work in place too, as you will feel guilty about putting something where it doesn't belong.

Another tip is: contain, contain, contain! Grouping items together by category and placing them in containers or decorative storage baskets not only keeps your space looking aesthetically pleasing, but it boosts functionality and saves time searching. Try to keep your containers matching in each room, whether they're fabric, acrylic or cardboard, as this will give a uniformed and stylish look. Consider the style and colour scheme of the space and use containers that will complement it. Don't forget to measure where the containers will go so you know they will fit.

When considering what type of storage boxes you need to contain your items, think about what is going to be stored in them and the space you have for the boxes. For example, you may want to contain items in a bits and bobs drawer – these will likely need shallow drawer dividers (see page 32). These come in all shapes and sizes so you can fashion the best set up for you and your drawers and what is going in them. Drawer dividers with sections are excellent for underwear drawers and bedside tables too.

Larger storage boxes are commonly used for children's toys, in bedrooms and in wardrobes. If you are struggling to decide what you will need for the items you have, always think about what they need to store and where the storage boxes are going as this will give you a better idea as to what kind of shape and size you will need.

top tip

You can never have enough containers and we definitely recommend buying more than you may need as you can always take them back. Not having them at the time can ruin your flow and finish. In this case, more is always best!

TIME FOR EVERYTHING TO GO BACK IN

Now everything is detoxed and contained in its relevant storage, it can be put back in place.

Really think about where everything is going to go. Consider practicality and your logic when you're in a rush and asking yourself: what do I use regularly and where do I use it? If they are items that you use every day, you need to make sure they are easily accessible. For example, if you like to get ready in the bathroom, then keep your make-up and toiletries in there. If you have a dressing table in your bedroom, keep these items there so when you get ready everything is easy to find – you want to waste less time scrambling around searching.

Items in the same category or group should be homed together. For example, stationery should all be kept in the same place, crafts could then also fall into this area too. Once items are grouped and going back in, keep items in their category and then colour-coordinate them. For example, in the wardrobe, group all denim together, knitwear together, then colour-coordinate within that category. This not only looks lovely but having items placed together helps you easily hunt out what you need and ensures you stay on top of your inventory – this applies to everything in your home.

ENJOY

Congratulations on your amazingly organised space! You can now enjoy all your hard work. You will now probably visit the newly refreshed area a few times just to marvel over your achievements! This is certainly our favourite part of a detox and organise. We take so much pleasure when showing our clients their newly organised space.

Now you have eliminated unnecessary 'stuff', you will have a better idea of what needs to live in that particular room, and you may feel it now needs a little revamp or a new piece of furniture. This is your chance to start making small, powerful style edits to give the room a new lease of life through the use of accessories or you may even be inspired to upcycle a piece of furniture, which could be as simple as changing the handles on a cupboard. For ideas and inspiration, see pages 188–211.

GIVE, SELL, GET RID? OUR TOP TIPS TO HELP YOU DECIDE

Once you have detoxed and assessed what you'd like to keep, you will still have the categories of leftover items that need to finish their journey. Here we take you through the options for how to deal with these and try to make sure they find the best possible new homes. Turn to page 44 for our handy flowchart if you're stuck on next steps and you'll soon discover which option is suitable for the item.

GIVE TO A LOVED ONE

Once you've completed your detox and you have your keep pile, consider whether you have any friends or family who would like or might use any pieces in good condition.

There is no better feeling than the gift of giving. Knowing a much-loved item has been given a new lease of life and gone on to be used by another person, especially a friend or relative, can be so rewarding. Items such as children's clothes and toys are always well received, or you could pass on books you've read for friends to enjoy, or even a perfume or beauty product you may not be fond of, but you think someone else may love.

GIVE TO CHARITY/DONATE

Donating items to charity enables you to pass them on knowing that they are going to be enjoyed by someone else and not just be thrown away or end up in landfill.

Before you decide to donate your items to a charity shop, check that they are clean and in good usable condition, not broken or badly stained – clothes and shoes need to have enough life in them to be resold and worn again. If they are badly damaged, they will need to be recycled or taken to clothing banks (check your local recycling centre). If you are donating games or puzzles, make sure that they contain all the correct pieces.

Double-check that the charity shop you are donating to accepts the items that you are donating, and they are happy to take them. Some charities, such as the British Heart Foundation, will come and collect furniture donations and offer free postage for donations up to a certain size/weight limit. Many charity shops have Gift Aid on donations so charities can make the most money possible (if you are a UK tax payer). Some shops like Oxfam also have schemes such as Tag Your Bag which gives you a membership number and card that's swiped with every donation. They then email you to say how much your donations have made when sold, which is epic. It's a wonderful feeling to give and it's heart-warming to know your pre-loved belongings are having a worthwhile impact.

SELL

Selling items that you no longer use gives you the opportunity to make money back from things that would otherwise be collecting dust!

If there are items you no longer want or need, local selling groups such as those listed on Facebook are an excellent choice as there are no fees and items often sell quickly to someone close by, which means they will be collected quickly too! There are also many reputable online selling sites such as Gumtree, Depop and eBay that are useful for reaching a wider audience. Pick the site that you feel is best suited to what you are selling. Look up similar items that other sellers are offering to get an idea of what you might be able to achieve pricewise. Also consider car boot sales, which are really good for selling older items that might be harder to sell online but still have some life left in them. If you are selling designer or vintage items, there are some reputable selling sites that are designed specifically for these items. A quick search online will bring up lots of options.

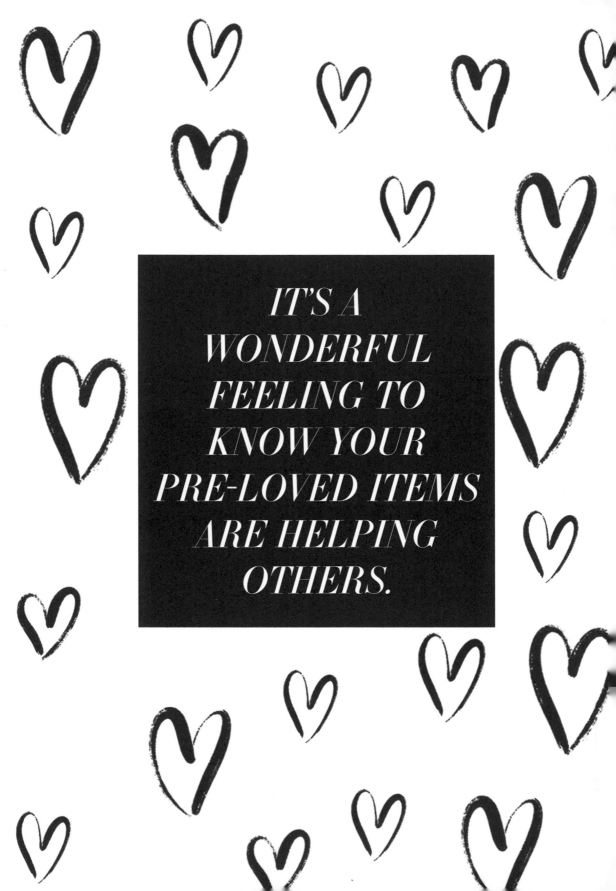

IT'S A WONDERFUL FEELING TO KNOW YOUR PRE-LOVED ITEMS ARE HELPING OTHERS.

RECYCLE

If an item has come to the end of its life and no-one has any further use for it, consider recycling it so it doesn't end up in landfill.

Look at what the recycling rules are in your area – you should be able to find this information online or you can ring your local council to check. Some items can be put out with your usual rubbish collection, but others may have to be taken to specific places, such as textile recycling banks for clothes that are too old or worn to be donated or regifted. For some items you can arrange a specific collection so they can be picked up and then recycled.

GET RID

There are some items that won't be be possible for any of the above options and you should discard them in as safe and environmentally-friendly a way as you can.

If they are broken or not made from recyclable materials, look at taking them to your local dump if they are too large to go out with your weekly rubbish.

GIVE, SELL, GET RID?

Our handy flowchart! If you're at a bit of a loss as to next steps for an item you're not keeping, try answering the questions below to work out the right direction for it.

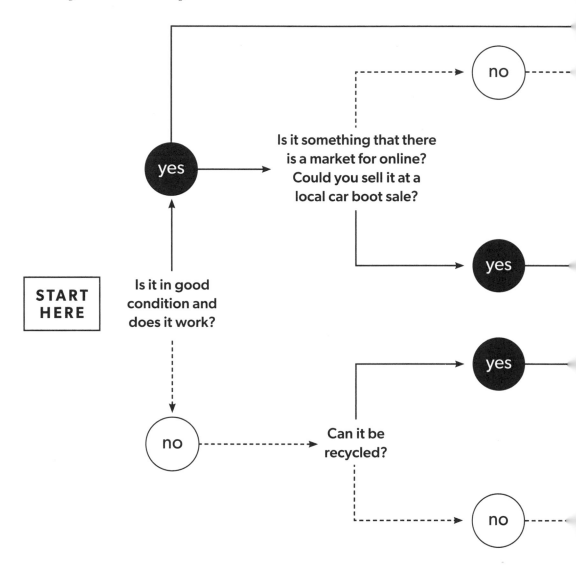

START HERE

Is it in good condition and does it work?

yes

Is it something that there is a market for online? Could you sell it at a local car boot sale?

no

yes

no

Can it be recycled?

yes

no

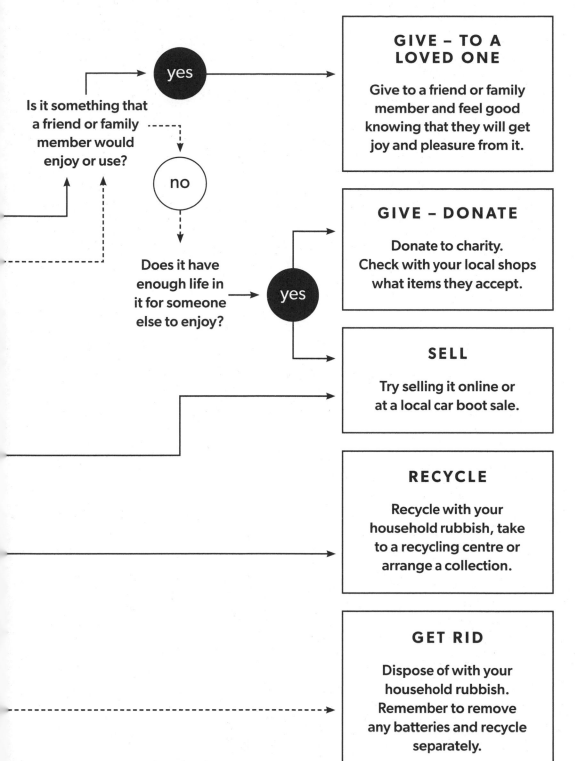

Is it something that a friend or family member would enjoy or use?

yes →
GIVE – TO A LOVED ONE
Give to a friend or family member and feel good knowing that they will get joy and pleasure from it.

no

Does it have enough life in it for someone else to enjoy?

yes →
GIVE – DONATE
Donate to charity. Check with your local shops what items they accept.

SELL
Try selling it online or at a local car boot sale.

RECYCLE
Recycle with your household rubbish, take to a recycling centre or arrange a collection.

GET RID
Dispose of with your household rubbish. Remember to remove any batteries and recycle separately.

Process

DETOX
and
ORGANISE

Now, you've got all you need
– let's work through your
home room by room

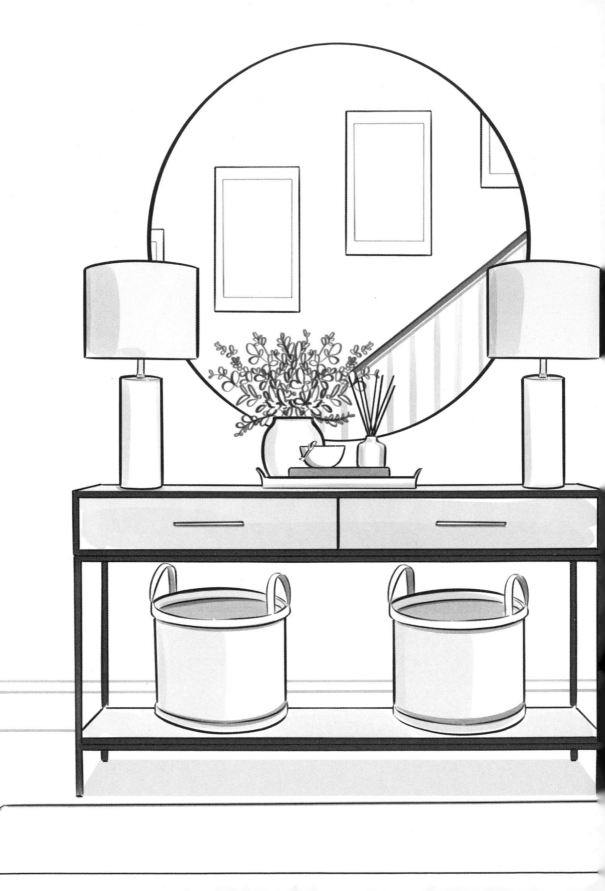

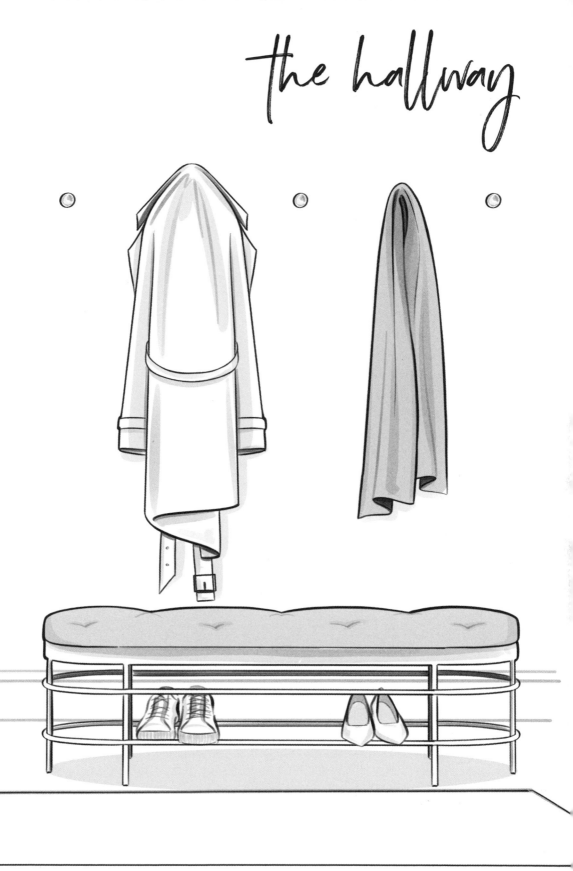

the hallway

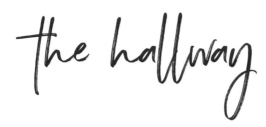

THE INTRODUCTION TO YOUR HOME

Besides the exterior of your house, the hallway gives the first impression of your home and provides guests with a glimpse of what is to come in the other rooms. It is often the most overlooked space; however, we think it's one of the most important.

We walk through the hallway throughout the day and it's the place where multiple items, including coats and shoes, happen to live, so it's definitely a space that needs to be carefully planned. Having a cluttered and untidy entrance will subconsciously make you feel chaotic the minute you walk through the door – it's the first view you see when you arrive and the last thing you see when you leave. It's vital to make sure people can travel through without blockages.

You want to set the overall tone and vibe from the moment you step over the threshold – your home is your sanctuary and when you arrive you should be greeted with calm. Stimulating the senses visually and through smell is a simple way to achieve this. Consider diffusers and candles in a scent that uplifts you and makes you feel happy (see page 208). This is the first thing your guests will smell when they arrive – there is great satisfaction in someone saying 'Ooh, something smells nice' when they enter!

Think about your daily habits. Your home needs to work with you, not against you, and you want to try to curate a space that is going to help make your life that little bit easier. There is no point designing something that doesn't suit your needs.

Organising and styling your hallway, as with any room, really all depends on the floor space you have to work with. The hallway can become a dumping ground for everyday items and can quickly evolve into a clutter hotspot; shoes scattered over the floor, shopping bags and deliveries stacked up by the door, and letters piled up on the side table. We've all been there!

Well, fear no more as we are here to help you create a clutter-free, calm and inviting space with our storage solutions and styling ideas. You will walk through the door and have an instant feeling of zen which will flow through the home.

Whether you have a large entrance or a small one, each can be streamlined and styled to suit you. It is important to remember that sometimes the area you have to work with and the items you need to home there aren't friends, so compromises need to be made. This doesn't mean you can't still make the most of the space and set the right impression from the get-go. We are going to list some common scenarios and give you inspiration for what you can do.

Firstly, you need to detox the space following the steps we laid out for you in The Process on pages 36–9. You don't want anything homed here that doesn't belong. So, first things first, empty the room and make a list of items that need to stay in the hallway and items that can be stored elsewhere. When you put together your 'need' pile think about it logically – the hallway is a space that takes you from the outside to the inside. Do you need to store coats and shoes in the hall? A bike? Pram? Post, umbrellas, keys, shopping bags and any other everyday items? Be ruthless yet realistic. Once you know what you have left to work with, you can then decide what you can use to style and organise the space.

Finding alternative homes for larger items can be difficult if you are tight on space or have no outdoor areas to home them. A garage would be the first place we would put bikes, scooters and perhaps your buggy or pram. If you don't have a garage, then a garden shed, or a garden storage unit, works well and there are smaller ones that fit on balconies to store items away outdoors but keep them protected from the elements. Once you have tackled these larger items that can be stored outside the house, it's time to work out what to do with the items that live in the hallway.

Whether you have a large entrance or a small one, each can be organised and styled to suit your life and needs.

The aim is for the space to be as clear as possible, creating a clutter-free zone.

We recommend the following items should stay in a hallway:

- ★ **umbrellas**
- ★ **coats** (if there is no other place to store them)
- ★ **everyday shoes** (if there is no space elsewhere)
- ★ **keys**
- ★ **candle or diffuser**
- ★ **storage baskets**
- ★ **rug or mat**
- ★ **footstool, ottoman or chair** (if you have the space)
- ★ **statement lighting or lamp**
- ★ **console table or sideboard**

Umbrellas can be stored in a simple umbrella stand or unit, or cupboard if there is space for one. If they are smaller umbrellas, then a storage basket is a perfect place to keep them on hand for when you go out.

If coats need to be stored in the hallway, make sure it's just a few everyday coats. You don't need your whole coat collection hanging up causing a big mass. You need to be able to find what you're looking for and use regularly at speed when you're in a rush. Hang them on a coat stand, hanging rack or on decorative pegs to make them look more stylish. Coat pegs should also be clear enough to allow guests to hang up their coats and scarves when they enter.

Shoes are handy to have in the hallway if you're constantly in and out of the house, but where possible store them away in a shoe cupboard so they're not in view or tidy onto a shoe rack.

The hallway is an obvious place to keep keys. However, do try to store them out of sight for security purposes. Decorative boxes are great to hide them away. Not only will this keep them safe, but by giving them a logical home, you won't ever lose them, we hope!

Storage baskets or boxes are an effective solution for a hallway to put away mail when it arrives and any other small items.

If you have the space, a runner rug or larger rug makes the space feel larger and will serve as a tool for pattern and detail, if your interiors are otherwise fairly neutral.

TOP TIPS for a stylish hallway

★ **NEUTRAL TONES TO MAXIMISE SPACE**
Choose neutral tones and colours – a simple yet effective colour such as a warm off-white will make the space seem larger and lighter.

★ **BE BOLD WITH A COLOUR POP**
Inject colour with an accent feature. If you like the idea of having a bold pop of colour but you're scared to decorate the whole hallway in that colour, try accessorising with bold vases, lamps, storage boxes or frames, or consider painting the inside of the front door – it will add personality to the space.

★ **ADD CHARACTER WITH WALLPAPER**
If you prefer the idea of wallpaper, choose something that will add character but not look too busy; if you have a smaller hallway and you're nervous to commit, start with the smallest wall first. You could use a geometric print, for example, and weave this accent around the home with accessories like geometric cushions or posters in frames.

★ **TRY A GALLERY WALL**
Large staircases or hallways are the perfect place to hang a gallery wall (see our top tips on page 201). This will add a personal touch as soon as you enter the home and will fill you with a warm fuzzy feeling of love and happiness from the photo memories or uplifting prints as you go up and down the stairs throughout the day!

★ **SHOWSTOPPING LIGHTING**
Choose a showstopping centrepiece to illuminate your hallway, especially if natural light is limited. Adding a striking feature light like a beautiful statement chandelier or large lantern will illuminate the space and is worth the investment as it will be one of the first things you will see when entering. It will sit as a key focal point for the area.

★ CLEVER CONSOLE TABLE

We love styling a console table that has drawers (see page 58) with trays and pots to keep items handy and easy to find when needed. Check out our guide to styling one on page 58, they're such clever bits of furniture, slimline and stylish, but super practical.

★ A TOUCH OF GREENERY

A simple orchid, a vase of fresh flowers or a modern pot with a large houseplant will make an instant statement in the hallway and will also bring life and oxygen into your home, not forgetting the added bonus of the fresh floral aroma that some flowers bring. (See page 206 for our favourite houseplants.)

★ STORAGE SOLUTIONS

Storage baskets or trunks are a genius way to hide clutter and items such as school bags, PE kits or shoes, which often get dumped in the hallway as soon as people enter the house. Post, deliveries and parcels can also be stored in baskets until they are opened and put in the right place. We find this is a common issue in our celebrity clients' homes. As they are being sent items on a daily basis it becomes so overwhelming that they just end up piled in the hallway. Popping them in a basket instantly makes the space appear less cluttered.

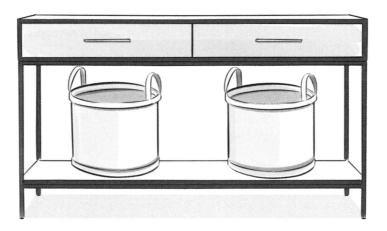

the small hallway

If you have a smaller hallway, you need to be a super smart with the layout.

A narrow hallway will benefit from having mirrors placed on the walls to bounce light and reflections. This will make the space appear larger than it actually is, not to mention give you the perfect opportunity to check your make-up before leaving the house!

A narrow shoe storage unit is an ideal way to house all your shoes when you're short on space. It can be dressed with a candle, flowers or plant on top.

A slim mirrored or glass console table can actually make the space appear larger and is perfect for hiding away items like keys and cash. People usually think placing furniture in an already small space will make it feel claustrophobic but it's actually quite the opposite (depending on the type of style used). Slim and airy furniture gives the illusion of not taking up much space while invoking the sense of having enough space to home a console table – it's quite clever! Choosing bulbous and chunky pieces won't work as well, so try to avoid these and focus on a balanced aesthetic.

A runner rug will add length to a walkway and can be vehicle for colour and texture that's lacking elsewhere. Always remember to go larger, as this will actually make the space feel bigger and more finished. When only a small part of the floor is covered, it will appear as though the rest of the floor has been forgotten about and draws your eye to too many different points instead of in one direction.

Under the stairs is an undervalued place in the home and it need not be, as there are plenty of practical storage options available and it's a way of taking advantage of an area that isn't necessarily used on a daily basis or on direct show. If it's more storage you're after, there are companies that build drawer spaces under the stairs which can then hold lots of items that would be cluttering the hallway area in an otherwise dead space. Or this space can be converted into a cupboard to home larger items such as bulky coats or cleaning supplies. If you live in a flat and don't have space under stairs, this is where you can make use of a hallway cupboard or clever console storage options.

Go floor-to-ceiling with slimline storage – using vertical space in a smaller hallway is absolutely essential. You can make a practical feature of a blank wall by turning it into storage – you can never have enough! Invest in wall-hung storage solutions such as shelves. If you're tight on space and you have a narrow hallway but tall ceilings, which is common in period-style properties, look into attaching units to the walls to keep clutter from the floor space. This will streamline the room and you won't be falling over items that are under your feet.

If storage isn't a requirement and you're just looking for ways to jazz up the space, you can use the tips above with the luxury of not having to worry about whether the item provides enough storage for your needs. You could even turn any space under the stairs into a library! See page 196 for our tips on styling shelves.

the large hallway

If you are lucky enough to have a large entranceway, you have more scope in what you can do to not only create storage but to style the space.

A larger area can accommodate chunkier items without them becoming too dominant. Consider a statement piece of furniture, like a console table, a round table or even decorative freestanding shelving which you can dress and style with candles, photo frames, vases and fresh flowers. Artwork is also a lovely way to fill wall space in a large hallway. The aim is to make the hallway as warming and inviting as possible upon entry.

A bench or footstool is another great piece of furniture to add to a hallway area. Hunt out those that can double up on a practicality level, e.g. a bench with plenty of depth for baskets underneath or a footstool with hidden storage, where you can put away unsightly shoes. Use these additions as ways to add bold pops of colour, either the fabric of the footstool itself or with neat cushions running along the bench.

When you have a large entranceway or even just high ceilings, it gives you the perfect opportunity to go big with statement lighting that will instantly add style and interest to the space (see page 53).

Coats are often the thing people find hardest to store if they have to be kept in the hallway. A coat stand can be a nice feature if you have the space for it – it can fill a corner of the room and offers that crucial practicality factor. Try not to overfill the stand as it can make the space look cluttered and messy. We also love a coat cupboard that can be home to all your coats without interfering with the rest of your wardrobe. Coats are often bulky and take up lots of space, so having them together behind closed doors is our favourite way of storing them. If you have the room, a statement wardrobe-style cupboard or an under-the-stairs cupboard can home all your bulky coats and any visitors' coats too. If you have cupboard space and no rail, consider adding hooks on the inside of the door to store coats out of sight.

Handy reminder: The Process

WHAT YOU NEED CHECKLIST

☐ bin bags

☐ vacuum cleaner

☐ cleaning products

☐ storage boxes/containers

☐ label machine/labels

The Style Sisters guide to styling your . . .

console table

If your hallway and table allows, add a pair of symmetrical lamps on either end – these will these give off a sense of balance and grandeur.

1. CONSOLE TABLE

Choose a console table that works with the style of your home. If you live in a barn conversion or cottage with wooden beams, consider a wooden table, or if you have a modern home, a metal or glass console would look great. If your hallway is smaller, try an acrylic or mirrored table to give the illusion of more space.

2. MIRROR

Adding a mirror to your hallway is a great way to open up the area to give a sense of more space, as mirrors bounce off light and reflection. If you don't want to hang a mirror, you could always rest one on the table against the wall.

3. LAMPS

If you like symmetry, you can place two lamps either side of the console table. Not only will it give adequate lighting, it also looks super stylish too. If you don't have space for two, one lamp works just as well. We love using lamps as a way of adding some height to your console table, however you can still get this effect by using any tall items, such as flowers, plants or decorative vases. This will give a stunning layered feel with different proportions.

4. VASES

Vases are a good way to add height to your console. Fill with flowers, foliage or houseplants to add a touch of greenery.

5. POTS/ACCESSORIES

Ideal for storing all those important bits and bobs you need before you walk out the door, such as keys, change and earphones.

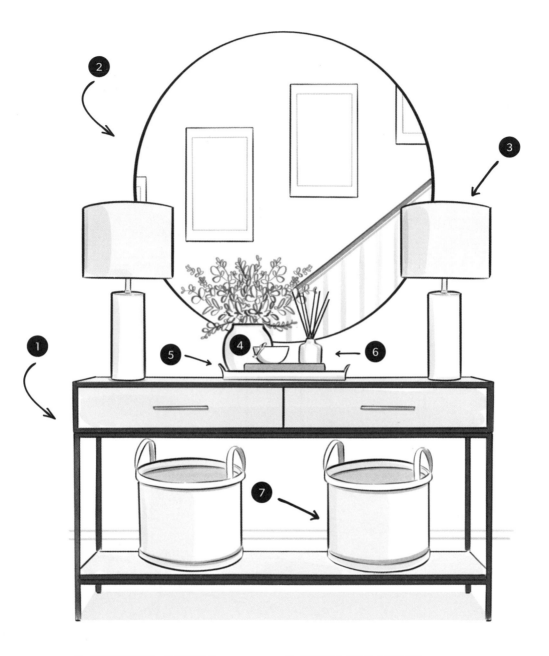

6. DIFFUSER, CANDLE OR ROOM SPRAY

Choose a refreshing and uplifting fragrance that makes you feel good as soon as you step through the door. It's the perfect way to welcome visitors into your home.

7. STORAGE BASKETS

A simple solution for keeping shoes, deliveries or post organised and tidy in one place.

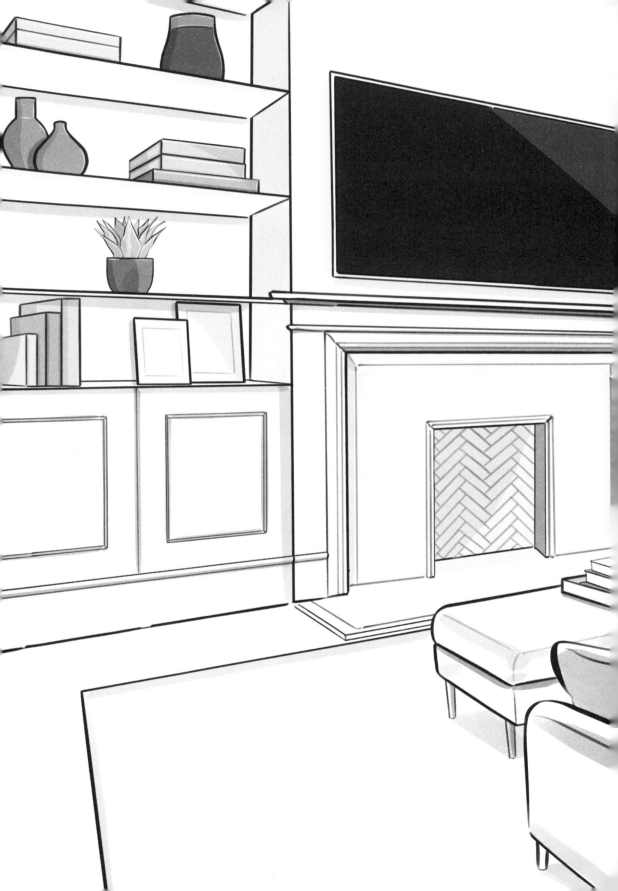

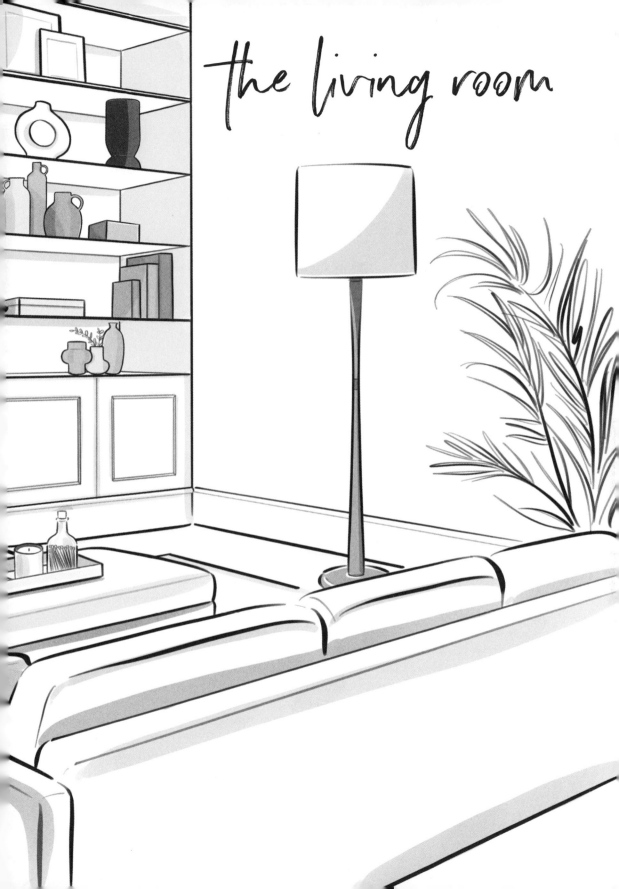

the living room

the living room

COMFORT & STYLE IS KEY

Your living room is the place you're likely to be when you want to chill out, watch TV and read, chat with family and friends and make beautiful memories. This room therefore needs to be clutter-free and inviting, with lots of warm lighting and soft furnishings. It should be a spot where you can switch off and recharge those batteries.

It's important to ensure this is a comfortable and functional room that you want to spend time in. It needs to look stylish, but it also needs to feel like your home. You shouldn't be worried about messing up the cushions or putting a drink on the side table.

To make the space feel balanced, place pieces of furniture on all sides of the room and try not to overfill one area with items as it will become off-balance and the room won't flow correctly.

Firstly, you need to detox the space following the steps we laid out for you in The Process on pages 36–9. Having a solid detox of items that no longer belong here will lead you to work out what you're using and what you're not using in this space. People tend to hold on to items such as board games they never play, DVDs they never watch, piles of outdated papers and magazines and bookshelves full of books that are just collecting dust. Scan the room and ask yourself what items haven't been touched in months or even years and what value they are adding. Your lifestyle may have changed – you may now have a young child and their toys to accommodate, priorities are always changing and you've got to make sure you overhaul your home alongside. For example, you may have shelves of old CDs or photos, which can now be transferred on to a computer or phone or put in your memory box.

The living room often has multiple uses and needs to be adaptable to modern lifestyles. Smaller houses, flats and homes with open-plan living may have the living room, kitchen, dining room and office all together in one large room. If not structured properly, this can feel very cramped and lack boundaries.

But you can flip these challenges on their head to make this type of highly functional space look larger than it is and super dynamic. This is also the case for expansively large living rooms, so they look like a well-loved home. It is integral to divide the room into different 'zones' or areas for its uses and to focus on flow and clear movement within it – for example, you have one zone for watching TV, one as your dining area and another for children to play in and one spot with your desk in, that you can tidy away at the end of a long day.

Devising separate zones within your living room for different functions will also work better for you and your family members' various needs. Many homes we have visited over the years have had lots of uses for the living area, but one common zone is a play area for young children – the amounts of toys children can accumulate over time is shocking! (We've both been there.) It's all about how you store or display them that is key. Having a zone dedicated to toys as opposed to having toys spread all over the room works far better, firstly because your child knows where all their toys are, and secondly because it doesn't make you feel like you're unwinding and chilling out in a child's play area when they go to bed!

With more people now working from home, there's also a growing need to divide the space into separate areas for living, relaxing and working. With no commute to separate the working day from the evening, people are looking for ways to maintain their work/life boundaries as it can be a struggle to transition from the frazzled working day to evening relaxation. Dividing your living space into distinctive zones for work and play will ensure it doesn't all blur into one and allow you that much-needed head space.

We recommend considering the room as a whole and making sure all the furniture is in sync so that it doesn't feel like a mishmash of styles. You can do this by choosing toy baskets in the same colour as other colours used in the room, making sure your table and chairs match the style and/or colour of your sofa and so on.

There are plenty of layout options for furniture, depending on the shape and size of the room; however, you must be realistic about what the space is mostly used for. If it's for chilling out with the family watching films and is a generally relaxed zone, then an L-shape sofa facing the TV is a great option. If your lounge is a formal space for entertaining and conversation, two smaller sofas facing each other is a better choice as it's more personal and encourages interaction. The larger the space, the more furniture you need to fill it. You may want extra seating to indicate different zones, i.e. a more chilled out area and then a formal space.

THE LIVING ROOM

SAMPLE STYLE SISTERS ROOM LAYOUTS

Before you start planning your room layout and zoning for an open plan area that needs to function as a living space/office/toy room/dining room etc, it can be really helpful to draw out the space of your room to get a room to get a vision of how things will fit together. Then you can get a rough floorplan in your head of how the furniture is going to flow and work in the space available. Here are some sample ones for you to spark a few ideas.

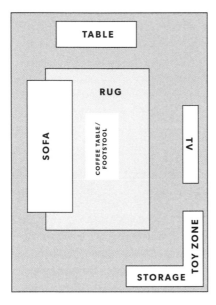

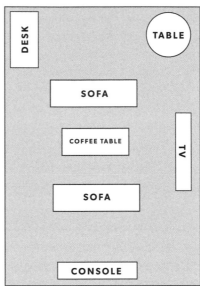

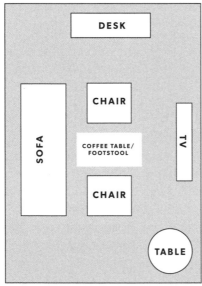

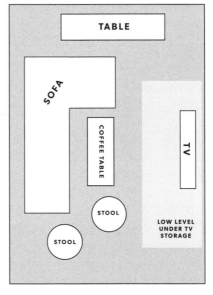

NOTES ON CURTAINS

Remember to go large and bold with the curtain pole and allow the curtains to be slightly longer so they drape on the floor rather than skimming the ground and coming up too short (this isn't a chic look).

Longer is better, but not too long... Just in the middle is just right! When choosing fabrics for your curtains and blinds, think about how long you're committing to them for, is it an impulsive, trendy purchase or are they a timeless, simple style? We tend to advise clients to opt for a neutral, plain or textured fabric as bold colours and prints can date quickly, and if you were to change the décor in your home it's a big expense to change all of the window dressings, whereas a neutral fabric will go with most interior styles.

how to...

HANG CURTAINS CORRECTLY

★ *Do position your pole approximately 10–15cm above the window (or go all the way to the ceiling).*

★ *Don't use a pole that is too short for the window, it must overlap the window opening.*

★ *Do get a pole that is long enough that the curtains don't cover up the window when they are pulled open.*

★ *Do measure your window properly to make sure you don't get curtains that are too short.*

★ *Do get curtains that reach the floor.*

TOP TIPS for a stylish living room

★ **SAVE SPACE**
If you are able to place your TV on the wall or above a fireplace, that's a big way to save space. Be careful not to place it too high on the wall, otherwise you'll end up with a stiff neck! It should be at a comfortable height that works with your sofa. We love using any available space for stylish storage – if you have a fireplace, making the most of the alcoves either side of it can add lots of storage with shelves or cabinets. You can also add a shelf above the fireplace for housing candles, frames and vases.

★ **CONSIDER COLOUR**
No matter the size of your living room, you can still be experimental with colour. People often think using dark colours on the walls will make the room appear smaller and darker, however this doesn't have to be the case if you keep the flooring, skirting, ceiling and doors lighter. Opt for light furniture too as it will complement and distinguish some gorgeous contrast in the space.

★ **WORK YOUR WALLS**
Whether you decide to have a gallery wall (see page 201), photos on sideboards or bookshelves, or statement pieces of art or poster prints, the lounge is the perfect room to inject your personality and personal touch. Matching your wall art to your accessories is a nice way to add colour without having to paint the walls. It also allows you the freedom to update the colour scheme quickly without having to do a complete redecorating overhaul.

★ **LIGHTING IS KEY**
A lot of lounges have spotlights, which can be great when you need lots of light but can be quite harsh if they're not dimmable. Adding lamps wherever you can makes for a relaxing atmosphere and from a practical angle, you'll create those cosy reading spots in a room. The curation of your space must align with the activities you'll be doing in it. Try to make sure all the lightbulbs give off the same type of light – warm, warm white or cool.

★ **WONDERFUL WINDOW TREATMENTS**

The right window treatment finishes the look of a room and a space can look unfinished if they are left bare (unless the room is ultra-modern with bifold doors or Crittall windows). Wooden shutters look striking from the outside looking in and are fitting in a period-style home with larger windows, you can have them open, half open or closed. Roman blinds are another fantastic option. We love a sheer blind underneath to give you privacy as it still allows light to flood the room. Curtains are a fab way to add drama, texture and luxury to a room.

★ **FEATURE FIREPLACE**

If you're lucky enough to have a fireplace, then make it a feature in the room. Traditional fireplaces in period-style homes are a natural focal point, while electric, streamlined fireplaces are neat and stylish, adding a contemporary feel. If you have a fireplace but don't want to use it for a real fire, consider tiling it with decorative tiles and placing logs, plants, flowers or candles inside. Log burners, which are increasingly popular as they come in so many sizes and shapes, will add warmth to your living space. These are a good solution as they can even be fitted if you don't already have a fireplace or chimney.

★ **SOFT, COSY FURNISHINGS**

There is nothing better than sitting back and getting comfy on the sofa and what better way than using soft, plump cushions and luxurious throws? Throws and blankets can be folded and placed on the arms of the sofa or in baskets stored away for when needed. Make sure they are soft and not itchy, and preferably washable in case of any spillages or accidents! If you have a footstool, consider folding and placing a throw over it, or a decorative footstool tray is stylish and practical.

★ **GO GREEN**

We love adding greenery to any room – plants bring life and oxygen to a space and a joyful pop of colour. You can opt for faux versions to achieve the same look without having to worry about the upkeep. If your room can take a large floorplant, we love a palm or birds of paradise plant. For a smaller room, orchids are a nice choice. (See page 206 for our favourite houseplants.)

★ **SET THE MOOD**

The lounge is the room you will be winding down in after a long day, so light a few candles or put your mist diffuser on to release a soft, calming fragrance. The soft glow will also produce a warm and relaxing light.

the small living room

Organising and styling a small living room can be tricky if there isn't much space for storage, so it's best to work out from the get-go what items are essential to make the room streamlined, practical, yet beautiful and homely.

Less is more in a smaller living room – you want to be able to add personality and style, but you don't want it to appear cluttered and messy. This is why we insist on the detox process to begin with. When you have less space you want to make sure you're not holding onto unnecessary items for no good reason.

When picking out items of furniture, consider if they can be used in different ways, e.g. a chair that can be used as a desk chair if working from home, a small gate leg dining table that can be used as a desk, a desk that can be turned into a side table or a decorative stool that can be used as seating or store toys or extra blankets inside. Foldaway furniture is a clever way to save space. Cluster side tables that sit inside each other give you two or three tables inside one main table, so you have the extra surface space there when needed for drinks or snacks.

If you have the space for a footstool to rest your legs on and stretch out while sitting on the sofa, and would prefer this option to a coffee table, a practical solution is to get a large tray that can sit on top of the footstool. This can then home decorative items such as coasters, coffee table books and magazines and any other daily items like TV remotes that you need within handy reach. This tray can be easily lifted from the footstool when needed and the solid straight base gives you somewhere to put a cup of tea or a glass of wine. You can even consider an ottoman footstool for extra storage.

Investing in a storage wall unit or bookcase will not only give the illusion of space, but it will home a lot of items, making it a purposeful addition. You can dress the shelves with photo frames, candles and vases to add personality to the room. Go up vertically with shelving into 'dead' space wherever you can.

Try adding transparent surfaces, such as a glass or mirrored coffee table. These will trick the eye into making the room appear larger as they aren't a solid block colour, which will appear heavier and denser in the room. It's best to avoid overfilling the floorspace to the point where you can't move freely. Mirrors placed around the room will boost light and reflections and will make the space appear larger.

In a small living room, it's important to keep the space bright and bounce light around where you can. You can do this easily by using light window dressings as darker curtains or blinds can prevent the light from flooding in and make the room look dark. Of course, some smaller lounge spaces can look amazing when made dark and moody, if this suits your style. Choose darker paint and window dressings for a cosy, dramatic vibe perfect for a cinema-style lounge area or snug-style room.

Eye-level lamps are a simple focal point. For a reading corner or chair, think about a floor lamp with downward lighting to illuminate the book or paper and make reading a comfortable experience. If you add a pendant ceiling light, remember to make sure that the glare doesn't interfere with watching the TV from the sofa, especially if the TV is mounted on the wall. Work out the lowest height the light can be at without obstructing your viewing. Try including long slim floor lamps that will take up less valuable square footage, but still add ambience.

Making a focal point in the room, whether it is a large piece of artwork or a tall houseplant in the corner, draws the eye to that point in the room, distracting from the actual size of the space.

Go large on a rug! The larger the better as it will make the room feel bigger and ground it as a whole. Make sure it sits under your sofa(s) and furniture as you don't want it looking like a little floating island in the living room sea.

the large living room

When we go to clients' homes, they often have expansive lounges but they never use them as they're always in the kitchen diner area as it's sociable and inviting. Again, splitting the room into zones for different uses is a great way to utilise a larger space and provides smaller, cosier areas to curl up and relax in.

If you have a long and narrow lounge, it can sometimes be challenging when trying to lay out furniture. Zoning is a simple way around this. Divide the room into two or three sections depending on the size of your lounge. Try pulling all your seating together in a sitting area to direct a main focus in the room. You will be amazed how this will immediately transform its functionality. Try using a sofa, table or rug to help define the smaller zones you have created.

Finding storage solutions for a larger lounge is easy – you can add sideboards which can home DVDs, books, toys and games. A feature bookshelf will add character to the room. Arrange books in height order or colour-coordinate them to make a stylish focal point. An open freestanding shelving unit can help to divide a room into different areas, and the shelves can be used for display purposes and zoning while still giving the illusion of space. Turn to page 196 for our guide on styling bookshelves.

Consider adding wooden panelling to the room. This is a beautiful idea for any home and will add luxury, a sense of height and clean lines. This is recommended if you're planning on painting your walls instead of using wallpaper. If you have a period-style home, also consider adding coving or other timeless classics like ceiling roses.

Handy reminder: The Process

TO-DO CHECKLIST

The following can be applied whether you are tackling an area at a time or completing the whole room at once!

- ☐ **Get everything out** – empty every cupboard!
- ☐ **Detox** what is no longer serving you
- ☐ **Categorise** all items
- ☐ **Assess the space** and consider purchasing storage boxes or storage furniture
- ☐ **Work out the best layout** for you and what's staying
- ☐ **Contain** your 'keep' items, label and put away

WHAT YOU NEED CHECKLIST

- ☐ bin bags
- ☐ vacuum cleaner
- ☐ cleaning products
- ☐ storage boxes/containers
- ☐ label machine/labels

The Style Sisters guide to styling your . . .

coffee table

The coffee table often takes centre stage in the living room, so it's important to keep it neat and interesting but also functional. Think of your coffee table like a piece of art – a visual statement made by creating a look of balance, style and personality.

There is no right or wrong when it comes to styling a coffee table, but there are a few guidelines you can follow to help make it a bit easier. Have fun and experiment – it's all part of the styling process, and if you get bored over time you can change it up a bit by swapping flowers or plants, shuffling around the books or adding a new a new object aligned with the changing season. This way you'll never get bored of the set-up you create.

Consider the proportions of the items on the coffee table – they should be the right size, not too big that they take over the whole space and not too small that they get lost. They shouldn't overwhelm the space or get in the way of its function. You still want to be able to place items, drinks or the remote control on the coffee table as it's a working piece of furniture that is essential in the room. If you're a big fan of symmetry, always remember the magic number of three! The middle object will ground the display, so this could be a vase of flowers and then on either side place a pile of books with a candle on top. Try mixing up heights and proportions within the three objects.

1. STATEMENT ORNAMENTS OR VASES

Find a key piece that will bring some interest and adds personality to the coffee table through colour, pattern or texture.

2. PLANTS

Houseplants are a great way of bringing life into a room. Consider smaller houseplants for your coffee table such as cacti and succulents. Choose a plant pot that complements your colour scheme.

3. CANDLES AND ROOM SPRAYS

The perfect way to set the right ambience in the room, from the scent to the warm, calming glow of a candle.

4. COFFEE TABLE BOOKS

Choose coffee table books that work with the aesthetics of the room and that interest you, they can also be a great conversation starter. No coffee table is complete without a selection of coffee table books, remember odd numbers work well.

5. DECORATIVE DISPLAY BOXES

Boxes are a perfect way to hide remotes and items like matches that need to be stored away.

6. DECORATIVE BOOK STAND

Add a decorative book stand to display your books open on the coffee table. You can open at your favourite page and change up every now and then.

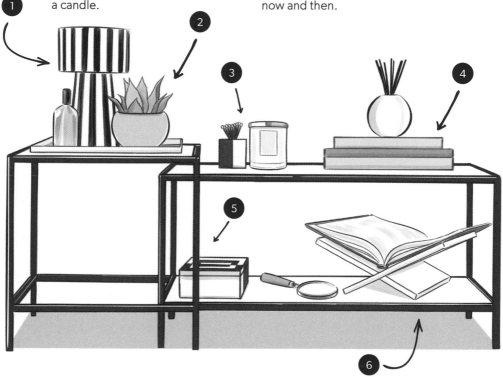

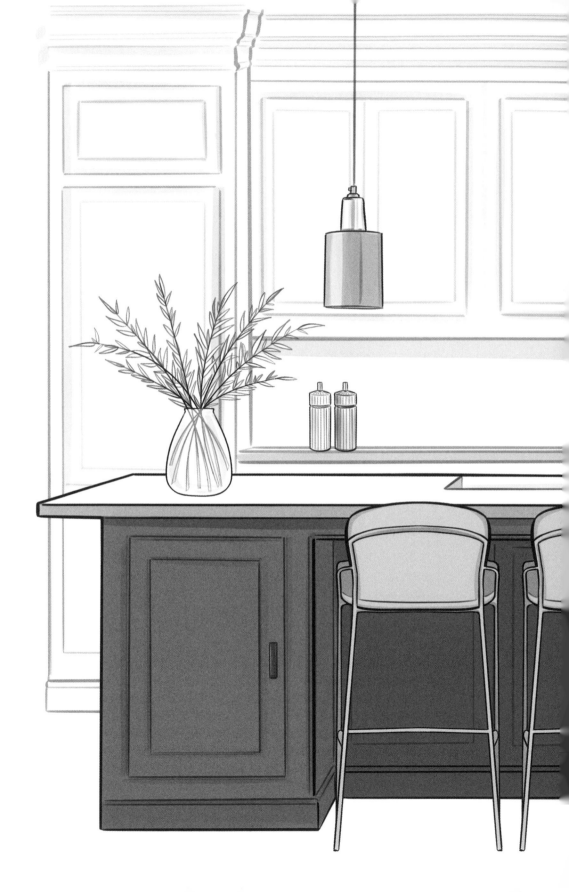

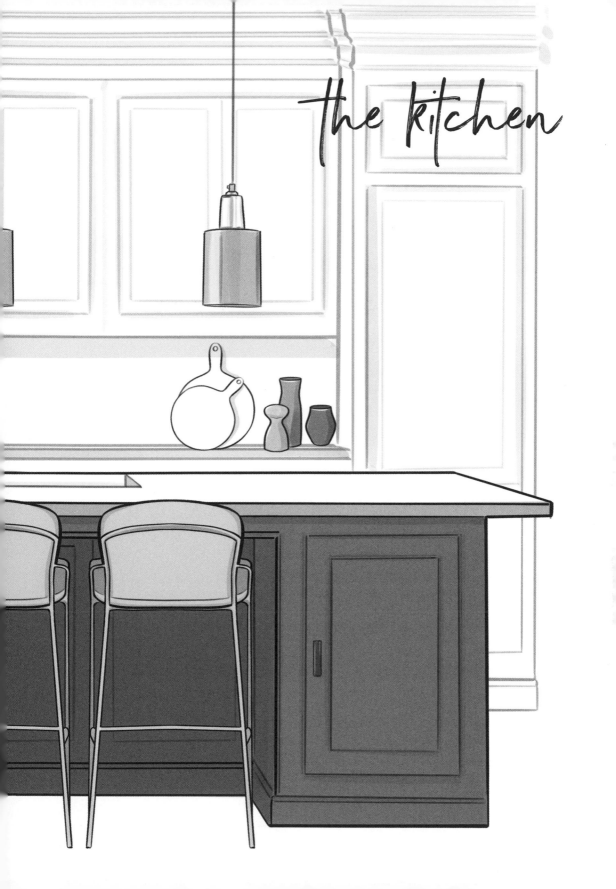

the kitchen

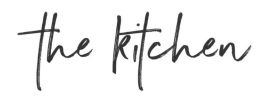

THE HEART OF THE HOME

The kitchen is usually the room where everyone gathers to eat, drink and chat. Whether you're entertaining guests, the neighbours have just popped over, or you're hosting coffee mornings with friends, the kitchen is a congregation point, where the hustle and bustle happens, and so it needs to be a clean, organised and inviting as well as functional space.

Kitchens are one of the rooms that vary the most from home to home. From a smaller kitchen in a flat to a large open-plan space with a dining area or breakfast bar, whatever sized room you are dealing with, we have the tools to make the most of your space.

To be clever with the areas that you have in your kitchen, you need to have a really good detox of all the items stored in the cupboards and drawers. This is key to making sure you're only finding homes for items you love and use. Space is valuable; you don't want items you never use taking it up!

Start with The Process we laid out on pages 36–9. When starting the detox, you really have to commit and be prepared for the space to get messy before it gets tidy. The kitchen is a big job but it's such a rewarding one and one that, once done, will make you feel back on top!

Start by getting everything out. And, yes, we do mean EVERYTHING. Check the dates on any food – are there food items that you know you're not going to eat? If so and they are still in date, you can donate them to your local food bank. When detoxing the cupboards and drawers, ask yourself: do you really need nine wooden spoons? Are you holding on to chipped mugs that you next to never use? Get ruthless and be realistic – will you ever use the fondue set that Auntie Tina gave you four Christmases ago?! Or you may have a sushi-making set gathering dust like our celebrity client Billie Faiers. Like her, you may have the best of intentions about using something, but truthfully know you never will.

There are often bulky kitchen gadgets that take up a lot of space that people have but never use, such as mixers or juicers or even make-your-own pasta machines (I mean, we wish we were that person, but we will never be that person!). Getting rid of these is an easy way to free up space, and if they're still in good condition, consider selling them or gifting them to foodie friends who will enjoy them. Be honest with yourself about what you're actually going to use or whether you're just holding on to an item because you like the idea of using it.

KITCHEN DETOX CHECKLIST
This is a list of common kitchen items you may be unnecessarily doubling up on:

★   wooden spoons
★   cutlery
★   mugs
★   plates, side plates and bowls
★   flasks/water bottles
★   **Tupperware** – make sure all boxes have lids and get rid of any that don't
★   kids' cutlery
★   pots and pans
★   place mats

PANTRY PERFECTION

Save space in the kitchen by taking items out of their packaging and putting them in smaller bags or decanting into jars – remember to label them with the best before date or remove and store cooking instructions with them in case you forget. We had a client who had about ten different herbal teas and she was tight on space, so we took the teabags out of each box, placed them in sealable bags and cut out the front of the box with the type of teabag on it and placed it inside the bags. We then placed the ten bags in a box with a lid that shut – it saved SO much space, going from ten boxes to one larger box. How simple is that!

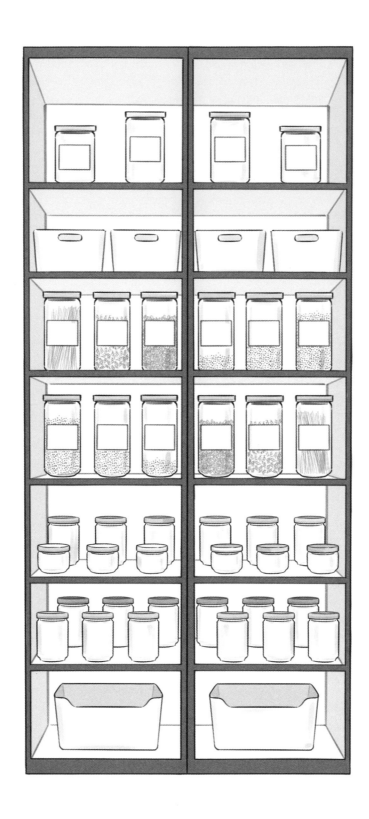

We love buying matching storage jars in different sizes to create this pantry-looking cupboard.

We've received thousands of amazing comments from posting our kitchen and pantry makeovers and the good news is it's an easy thing to do in your own home and gives a wow factor to your kitchen. Try to keep jars matching – this will nail the clean, clear aesthetic! We recommend picking a style of jar that comes in lots of different sizes as they are perfect for pastas, grains, spices, sweets, chocolate and all the dry goods in the kitchen.

You can make or purchase labels and label each jar with what's inside. This makes ingredients easier to find and looks super stylish, especially on spice jars. You can also get stackable jars and containers, which not only help you to keep certain items together, but also allow you to maximise space. These containers ensure you utilise the maximum height of the cupboard which would otherwise be dead space. This is especially handy in smaller kitchens. When putting everything away, group similar items together. You want your cupboards to make sense. For example, condiments, spices and sauces all sit well together so these can be stored in the same place; tins and jars should stay together; sweets and goodies in the same cupboard and so on.

top tip

Don't forget to add when items go out of date. Using the label machine, type out the best before date and place on the bottom of the jar/container to remind you when to chuck it and refresh.

UNDER THE SINK

Under the sink can become a dumping ground for cleaning products and cloths. As with most messy cupboards, you end up losing track of items you already have and so buy the same thing again, wasting money as a result. But it doesn't have to be this way as organising and streamlining this area is straightfoward and won't take you long at all – a perfect example of a doable task that will put you more in control. Investing in under-the-sink caddies or units that are designed for this type of cupboard adds storage space around the sink pipes. If you have a drawer or small cupboard under the sink, add containers where all items can be kept together. If you don't have space under the sink for a caddy unit, consider running a tension rod across the cupboard from left to right and then hanging your cleaning products off the pole. This way you're making the best use of the open space in the cupboard. You can also purchase containers that stick to the inside of cupboard doors. These can store sponges, cleaning cloths or bin bags.

top tip

Group items into containers by category. This helps you keep the space organised and ordered.

If you are guilty of purchasing multiple products and having overstock, think about if you have anywhere else in the home, such as a spare cupboard, garage or utility room, where they can be stored until needed. You only want the essentials under the sink – washing up liquid, antibacterial spray, cleaning products, laundry detergent and dishwasher supplies, if you have one. We love decanting our cleaning products into clear containers and adding a simple label so that they look stylish if displayed on a shelf.

LOCATION, LOCATION

When organising your kitchen, think about the items that you use on a daily basis as they will need to be easily accessible and within easy reach when you're cooking and working in the kitchen. We like to keep anything hot-drink-related above or next to the kettle or near the boiling water tap, if you have one. Keep the mugs and hot drink supplies contained together in a cupboard or in cupboards next to each other as they will be used together. If possible, try to keep plates and bowls all together and place them near the oven in a drawer or cupboard. This way it's easy to access a plate or bowl when serving up food.

'I AM OBSESSED BY EVERYTHING THESE GIRLIES DO. THEY HAVE SO MANY SPACE-SAVING AND ORGANISING TIPS THAT YOU JUST DON'T THINK OF YOURSELF.'

Vogue Williams

It makes sense to store any cereals, bread, spreads and any other breakfast-type foods near your toaster and/or microwave. We like to keep condiments, herbs, spices and sauces near the oven, so they are easily accessible when cooking. You can then fill in the cupboard gaps around this and do what works for you and your space. Remember to gather the same category together, for example rice and pasta in the same cupboard, then snacks, crisps, cakes and chocolate all together in one place or all in a special spot out of reach.

DRAWERS DOS AND DON'TS

Dividing drawers into sections will make them more organised and it will be much easier to find what you're looking for. Cutlery trays are a must-have in cutlery drawers as they separate all the knives, forks and spoons and stop them all mixing together in a big mess. You can also get larger trays for organising bigger items such as utensils. Adjustable drawer dividers are amazing tools for zoning within a drawer. We know lots of this is common sense, but it is easy to forget and it takes thought and focus to get it perfect.

top tip

If you're tight on drawer space, you can group your utensils together in a stylish pot and place it next to your cooker for easy access, or consider rails over the cooker where you can hang them. The trick to keeping everything looking stylish and organised when having items on display is to have everything matching or co-ordinated. Make sure your utensils are all a similar style and work with the look of your kitchen; the same goes for any jars or pots. Having everything in sight doesn't always have to mean cluttered and messy!

Everyone needs a bits and bobs drawer! It can be any drawer (or cupboard) that works for you around the home, but it can often be found in the kitchen. It normally contains things like pens, Sellotape, scissors and matches or lighters for example; items that you need regularly but that you don't necessarily have an exact home for. The key to keeping this type of drawer organised is to contain its contents, and you can do this by using shallow drawer dividers for different items. Not only will it look cleaner and more organised, but it will be easier for you to find exactly what you need, when you need it!

Batteries are found in this type of drawer, but did you know that these need to be stored safely? There are battery containers available to buy where all the different sized batteries have their own section, as it is dangerous to store batteries of varying voltages and sizes together as it can be a fire hazard. We probably shouldn't advertise it, but it was in the early days of our Style Sisters journey that we discovered this! We had been documenting a client's kitchen detox and organisation on Instagram and we were organising her batteries together into a drawer. While it looked lovely and organised, we later discovered that different battery types need to be kept separately. We didn't realise until we had left her home and looked at our phones. We had received loads of messages from people about how batteries shouldn't be stored together as it can cause a fire! Safe to say we both panicked and felt horrendous about it. We called the client immediately and held our hands up. Thankfully she was more than understanding and said she had never heard that before either, so everything was OK. Phew!

STORING MEDICINE

Housing important medicines and first aid kit in the kitchen makes total sense. If you do, always remember to put them high up out of the reach of children and away from any cupboard that gets hot.

We like to store everything from paracetamol to plasters together in one basket or box, so that it's all in one place. This is especially helpful with medicines stored up high as it allows you to see what you have without anything getting forgotten about at the back of the cupboard! When detoxing the kitchen, remember to check the dates on all your medicines as this important detail can be overlooked.

top tip

If you have the space, you could store any children's medicine separately from adult versions to save time sorting through when you need something quickly.

TOP TIPS for a stylish kitchen

★ **COLOUR PALETTE**

The colours used in a kitchen all depends on the look you're going for – you may opt for clean white and bright or Scandi hues or use it as your outlet for adding colourful signatures of personality, such as a bold kitchen island, brightly painted cupboards or funky bar stools. At Style Sisters, we do advise our clients to be careful about adding expensive bright and bold pieces. You might want a hot pink kitchen island this year, but are you likely to go off it in a few years' time? Rooms like the kitchen are an investment and it is best to use neutral colours and then accessorise with pops of colour and interesting metals for door handles if you want to boost vibrancy and character, but don't want to spend much.

If you have a small kitchen, keeping it light, bright and airy is an obvious option. However, if you do want to add darker accent pieces, then do so with chairs, stools or accessories on the worktops. If you have a larger kitchen with lots of space and natural light, choosing darker units and worktops is an option if moodier tones are more your style.

★ **WORKTOPS THAT WORK**

Making sure your worktops are functional for your day-to-day routine is very important, and having lots of items constantly out and cluttering up the space is not ideal as it can also make you feel mentally messy. Try to keep the worktops primarily clear apart from items that are frequently used like tea, coffee and sugar pots (or canisters). Chopping boards, decorative salt and pepper mills, and cooking oils are handy to have out ready to access when prepping and cooking food. Remember to keep ingredients looking pretty in decorative containers and keeping these matching and co-ordinated to help with the flow of the worktops. A decorative fruit bowl is an essential addition, not to mention a constant reminder to eat your five a day!

★ PRACTICAL LIGHTING

Your choice of lighting in a kitchen is dependent on the space and style of your room. Having bright lighting is important when prepping, cooking and eating food, but it's also nice to have the option of reducing the brightness of the lights when you're entertaining or enjoying dinner. The most popular style of kitchen lighting is spotlights and pendant lighting if you have an island. Pendant lighting placed over an island or dining table gives the room a special feature and focal point, and extra lighting over this area is handy when you're preparing food. Consider also using lights under the cupboards to give the worktops a soft glow and create an evening ambience. If you have a larger kitchen diner space, consider having wall lights and lamps as you can just use these and turn your main lights off when you want to increase ambience.

★ FAVOURITE FLOORING

Flooring in the kitchen has to be durable and withstand spillages and items dropping on it and be easy to clean. We commonly visit clients' homes and are confronted with two types of flooring in the kitchen area: wood and tiles. This can be an awkward thing to style around, so we advise our clients to run the same flooring running throughout the room for a continuous flow. Opt for flooring such as tiles, or LVT (luxury vinyl tiles). If you're having a kitchen renovation or building a kitchen from scratch, consider putting in underfloor heating to add an element of luxury, if it fits your budget.

★ HERB HEROES

If you fancy adding a little bit of greenery to your kitchen and bringing a bit of the outdoors in, adding small pots of herbs is one way to add a pop of life and colour to the space. They smell great and can be used in your cooking – fresh ingredients on tap!

★ ORGANISE YOUR SCHEDULE

The kitchen is normally the place where your calendars, invites, save the dates and school letters end up gracing the fridge or piled up on the worktops. Work out if this method of displaying your daily to-dos is right for your home. Consider investing in a magnetic blackboard or a pin board that can be placed on a wall or inside a kitchen door and used to organise your invites and write down appointments and meetings, etc. Remember it's all about having a practical yet stylish home that works for you and your lifestyle.

the small kitchen

You can make the most of a small kitchen by seeking out clever storage solutions and planning the design carefully. There are lots of fantastic options available depending on your space.

Pots and pans can take up precious cupboard space so consider placing a rail above the cooker and hanging them from that instead. You can attach a magnetic strip to the wall and store your kitchen knives on there to save drawer and/or counter space. Over-the-door kitchen organiser racks are also a great way to maximise space in an otherwise wasted area.

A Lazy Susan (a rotating round tray) is such a handy addition to your kitchen to place your must-have condiments, they take up minimal space but still give you plenty of storage and keep everything looking neat and contained.

A breakfast bar with stools is a simple solution to fit an eating area into a smaller kitchen that might not have room for a table and chairs. Or consider an extendible or foldable kitchen table that can also double up as a countertop when not in use. You can also get hold of tables that are freestanding or that attach to the wall and can then be folded down, only taking up space when in use. There are so many options that you are bound to find something that suits you and your home perfectly. Don't be afraid to think outside the box; the chances are someone's designed something that would work for your space. Pinterest is a creative place to get inspiration if you're feeling a little stuck.

top tip

To maximise space in a small kitchen try:

★ *Stackable storage baskets and storage baskets that can be added to the inside of cupboard doors.*
★ *Over-the-door storage racks.*
★ *Shelf steps for tins and herbs.*
★ *Pots for utensils that can be put on the worktop.*
★ *Floating shelves for cookbooks and plants.*

the large kitchen

A larger kitchen gives you more options, but it can sometimes also leave you feeling confused as to how to properly organise the space.

There are a few factors to consider when organising a larger kitchen: do you have a separate dining area? Do you want a TV and sofa seating area? How about a breakfast bar or a dining table? Or all of these? Having a kitchen large enough to accommodate all these different areas in one living space is the perfect way to create the hub of the home. This is especially helpful if you have young kids who you want to supervise while you're busy in the kitchen.

When dividing your kitchen into different zones consider how best to use the space. Have you got a spare wall to place a TV on? Is there room for a sofa or a couple of chairs in front of it? Can you rejig the current layout so you can have the space you have always dreamed of? You want this room to be social but functional too.

UTILITY ROOM/AREA

If you have a larger house, you might be lucky enough to have a separate utility room too. If not, the following advice can be applied to a utility area in your kitchen to try to keep the space streamlined. If your utility room is home to your washing machine, tumble dryer and laundry items, it's a great space to get super organised in and order your supplies.

BE SPACE SAVVY

As with the rest of the kitchen, you need to be space savvy with any cupboards and shelves by using slick containers and clever storage ideas. Use every bit of space possible – stack storage boxes on top of cupboards if there is room and use strong ones with handles (IKEA or iDesign both stock options) so it's easy to reach up and grab them when needed. Don't put items you use every day in these but utilise them for overstock or items that you need occasionally, such as party plates, fondue kits, extra mugs.

The insides of cupboard doors can have hooks for tea towels or cloths, or use shelves with sticky backs to hold items such as cleaning products or dishwasher or washing tablets. Make sure the cupboard door can shut before you stick it on, an easy error to make!

We always find that removing packaging and decanting items is a simple hack to gain a surprising amount of space. Often items are packaged in larger boxes to protect them and by taking them out you will find yourself with more room to work with. When removing items from the packaging, make sure the containers you place them in are childproof in case your little one gets their hands on them. Dishwasher and washing tablets are toxic and can be dangerous if swallowed. Storage with airtight locks or clips work well, or place containers high and out of reach of small hands.

When buying storage for the kitchen, utility room and bathroom, make sure the containers can be wiped clean in case they get food or liquids on them – stained fabric boxes won't look or smell very nice once they get dirty!

LOVELY LAUNDRY

If you have space for laundry bins for different coloured laundry, this is a great idea. Have three containers – one for lights, one for darks and one for mixed – and this way you can keep an eye on the washing building up and wash items more efficiently.

Keeping an ironing board in the utility room is handy as it means it doesn't take up valuable space elsewhere. If you have a tall cupboard, think about placing the ironing board in there so it isn't just leaning up against a wall. If you don't have a big cupboard, consider hanging it from a hook on the back of the door, the same goes for a freestanding washing line or heated rail.

ASSORTED STORAGE

Vacuum cleaners tend to be an item that our clients have a nightmare storing, so we recommend storing them out of view in the utility room or under the stairs in the hallway. If you don't have that luxury and it's a small hoover, then hang on a clip on the wall or back of a door. The utility room is a good place as they can be plugged in and charged if they are portable.

A utility room is also a good place to store wellies and shoes. If you have a sink in there, this is great for cleaning kids' football boots or wellies after a forest walk. If you have pets, we recommend storing their pet food and supplies in the utility room. This way they are out of the main cooking and food area of the house, they're all contained and stored in the same area, and are easy to find for you and your family.

Handy reminder: The Process

TO-DO CHECKLIST

☐ **Detox** cupboards and drawers

☐ **Check** sell-by dates

☐ **Categorise and group** similar items together

☐ **Decant** anything that can be transferred into canisters

☐ **Take items out of packaging** to create more room

☐ **Use** storage containers to keep everything looking neat and organised

☐ **Assess the space** and work out the best layout for you and your kitchen

☐ **Put everything away**

☐ **Enjoy!**

WHAT YOU NEED CHECKLIST

☐ bin bags

☐ vacuum cleaner

☐ cleaning products

☐ storage boxes/containers

☐ label machine/labels

☐ drawer dividers

Top Tips
for updating your . . .

kitchen

If your kitchen is looking a little sad but you don't want to splash out on a whole new kitchen, here are a few hints and tips on how to update and create a stylish space:

1. DECORATIVE DOORS
Update the kitchen doors by painting them. You can get them professionally sprayed or use a hard-wearing kitchen cupboard paint and primer to instantly create a whole new kitchen look! Make sure you clean the doors with a sugar soap scrub to remove any excess oil and dirt before painting.

2. CHANGE THE DOORKNOBS OR HANDLES
This is an inexpensive and quick way to update your kitchen.

3. TOP TILES
Are your tiles looking a bit drab? Is the grout looking grubby? Then paint them with some tile paint. This will make the kitchen appear fresh and new.

4. ACCESSORIES
Purchase new and matching accessories for the worktops, such as soap dispensers, vases and chopping boards.

5. PAINT JOB
Painting floor tiles with floor paint can give a kitchen a new lease of life.

'THESE GIRLS ARE AMAZING. THEY'VE HELPED ME WHEN I NEEDED IT MOST. WHETHER IT BE MOVING INTO A NEW HOME OR JUST WHEN LIFE GETS ON TOP OF YOU. THEY ARE ABLE TO MAKE YOU FEEL LIKE YOU'VE GAINED BACK THAT LITTLE BIT OF CONTROL INTO YOUR LIFE WHEN YOU'VE LOST IT. KIND, CARING, STRONG WOMEN THAT WE NEED IN THIS WORLD.'

Stacey Solomon

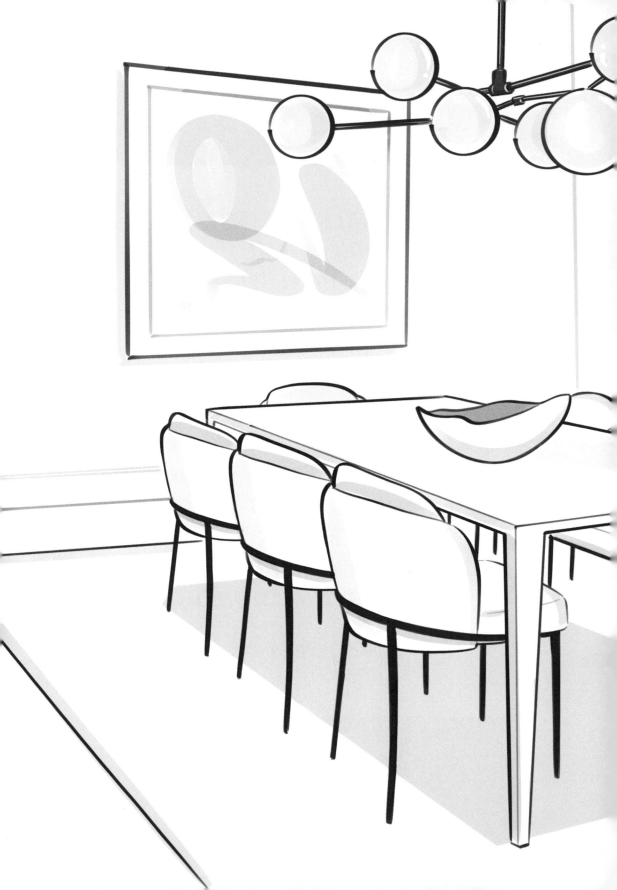

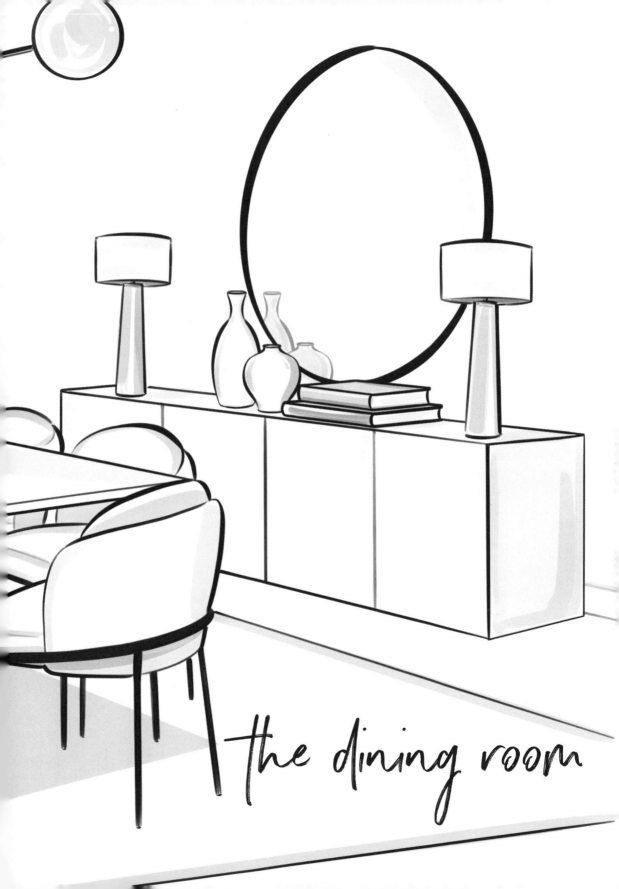

the dining room

the dining room

EAT AND ENTERTAIN TO
YOUR HEART'S CONTENT

A dining room is defined as 'a room where meals are eaten', but in reality
it can serve so many purposes in your home. You might have a whole room
for dining which may only be used for dinner parties or special occasions
throughout the year like birthdays and Christmas. Or your 'dining room'
could be part of another room in the house like the kitchen or living room,
it may even function as an office in the day. The following hints and tips
can be applied to your dining area regardless of its size or wherever it may
be in the home.

First things first, it needs to feel inviting and a place where you want to spend
time to eat, chat and entertain. This is a chance to design a super social space
that can cater to all the ways in which you want to use it. We know that small
spaces can be a challenge around the home, and this can definitely be the
case with a dining room. You might initially think that you don't need to
store too many items here; however, once you've got everything out you will
probably be surprised by how much there is to detox.

As with every room, start with getting all your items out to see what you're
dealing with. Follow The Process on pages 36–9. You'll probably have a
selection of napkins, tablecloths, table runners, alcohol, glasses, plates, cutlery,
games, books… You can find alternative places around the home for these
items if space is an issue; however, these items work well if there's room for
them to be kept in the dining area. It makes sense for these things to be homed
where they are going to be used and are easily accessible.

STORAGE SOLUTIONS
Think about the seating area where your table is – could you use a built-in
bench with under-seat storage? This could be with a lid that lifts or that
includes drawers, and then you just need to pad out the top of the bench
and add cushions to make it comfortable. This way you are creating a
multipurpose piece – storage and seating – win–win!

If you have a corner or alcove in a wall, place a side unit or dresser in the space or add shelves and decorative storage boxes to act as drawers. You can use each basket or container as if it is a section in a cupboard or drawer.

If you want something a little more bespoke or have an irregular-shaped wall, then finding off-the-shelf furniture might not be easy. Consider commissioning a carpenter to buld a beautiful piece of furniture that perfectly fits your space – it will be worth the investment and last for years to come. You can never have too much storage space and this can often be a real selling point if you choose to move.

WHAT GOES WHERE

We recommend having a sideboard or cupboard with drawers to home items that you will need for hosting and dining. If you like to keep your fancier plates, cutlery and glassware for when guests come over, it's a good idea to keep them separate from your everyday pieces, so they won't be taking up prime space. This also prevents them from getting damaged.

Napkins, napkin rings, tablecloths and runners can be stored in a drawer or storage box. They are probably not going to be used every day, so putting them all in the same place means they can be found quickly and easily.

We love to store board games and after-dinner games in a sideboard near the dining table so they're within easy reach to play after a delicious meal. Having guests over and enjoying some nice food and drink and playing games is our perfect night in.

Consider commissioning a carpenter to build a beautiful piece of furniture or shelving that perfectly fits your space.

THE DINING ROOM

If you have a certain way you like to decorate or arrange your dining table, it's a good idea to store everything for that look or colour palette together, such as the tablecloth, candles, napkin holders, etc. If you have tablewear that is only ever used for Christmas and you are short on space, put it away with your other Christmas decorations. It doesn't need to be taking up valuable space in the dining room all year round.

If you like the idea of having a home bar area, consider using a sideboard to store and/or display alcoholic drinks, glasses and any cocktail kit. Or for something a bit more decorative, try a drinks trolley which will add a bit of style and fun to your home and is perfect for mixing up after-dinner cocktails!

Alternatively, if you don't have space for a piece of furniture, wall shelving can also be a great spot for a mirrored drinks tray, to house all your special glasses and spirits and make a beautiful, simple feature as long as it doesn't get too cluttered.

Categorising your drinks trolley stops it from looking messy and cluttered. Try grouping glass types together and make sure you separate wines and spirits. If you don't have room for a trolley, small drinks trays on shelves can also look really special.

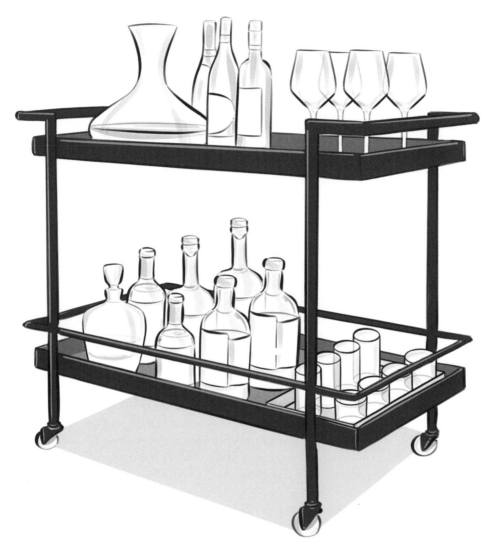

top tip

If you want to have a seriously organised-looking trolley, put spirits into matching decanters.

TOP TIPS for a stylish dining room

★ **ADD ART**

Hanging interesting artwork on the dining room walls will add personality and can become a great talking point when you entertain guests. We love to add wall lights that can sit above the artwork too. They give a really luxurious vibe and can also be perfect if you want to create some mood lighting in the room.

★ **COLOUR POPS**

Try adding colour to the dining area. If you have a large dining room, it can easily hold a dark, rich colour on the walls or just one feature wall. Deep navy, dark teal and dark grey all look lovely in a dining room, especially if you get a lot of light in that space. If you prefer to stick with safer neutral colours, then a soft warm greige, off-white or a monochrome theme works well, and you can then add bolder, darker furniture to complement the paler tones.

If you want to inject a bit more personality with brighter colours, this can be done through artwork, table décor, napkins or a floral display in the room. Whether it's on the walls or accessorising with a colourful table, adding a pop of colour to what can sometimes be quite a bland space will transform the room. It will be one of the first things you and your visitors notice when they enter.

★ **TOP TABLES**

The standout piece in nearly all dining rooms will be the table you sit around to eat and enjoy your food. There are so many different styles and shapes of dining tables, so think about the shape of the room and work out if a round/oval table would work better than a square or rectangular one. Avoid huge, chunky tables in smaller spaces that will overwhelm the room - opt for multi-functional pieces.

If you're tight on space, a round table might work best as you won't have any sharp corners to bump into.

If you have young children, glass or gloss tables are sadly a bit of a no-no as they can easily get scratched and marked and then look ruined and old in no time. Not to mention that cleaning young children's fingerprints off a glass table will become your worst nightmare and a game you will quickly want to quit! A wood, marble or varnished table will work better, is much easier to wipe clean and is far more practical.

If your children are older or it's an adults-only zone, we do love a glass dining table in smaller spaces as to the eye it seems to take up less space in the room.

top tip

Any table can be transformed with a lovely linen tablecloth or table runner. This will instantly update your table and will look more formal, especially for special occasions.

★ **CHOOSING CHAIRS**

Think about the durability of your dining chairs. Do you have children? Do you want to be able to wipe them clean if there is a food or drink spillage? If so, then a wipeable material like leather, wood or acrylic will be a better option for you. However, they are usually a bit harder and can become uncomfortable after sitting for a long time, so a padded and upholstered chair is a better choice if you're planning on hanging out around the table for a while. If you do have harder chairs, an easy solution is adding a seat cushion, or a fur throw for a little extra comfort and style. It's all about working out your needs and how you really use certain rooms in the house. You can then purchase items based on their practicality.

★ **TABLE SCAPING**

Some people like to have a formal table permanently laid with charger plates and/or place mats on the table, with plates and cutlery all styled as a decorative feature. If this isn't your style or you like a more minimal look, try a more contemporary centrepiece like a simple vase filled with flowers, dried pampas grass, greenery or even a tray with a few decorative items on like a candle, ornament and some long matches, which will also bring your table to life. The centrepiece for your table should never be a last thought. It can be a lovely way to bring the room together, so don't miss the opportunity to add a wow factor in the middle of the table.

★ **GO FOR A GALLERY WALL**

The dining area is an ideal place to add a gallery feature wall (see page 201). Filling your wall with lots of lovely memories or poster prints with quotes or images that inspire you and make you feel happy is a nice touch for where you eat and entertain, and will help inspire the happy vibes that you want around your home.

★ **LOW LIGHTING**

Lighting in a dining area is especially important – you don't want guests to feel like they have bright, unflattering spotlights interrogating them as they are eating at your table, but it shouldn't be so dark that they can't see what's on their plates. (Unless you're a terrible cook, in which case the room being dark could work in your favour!) You're ideally looking to create a warm, calm vibe. Dimmer switches are great as you can adjust the lighting to however bright you need it. If you already have spotlights, it's simple to swap dimmers in and you'll notice such a difference to the atmosphere of the room.

Think about the type of light you want. Are you going for a statement pendant that hangs over the table? These can look really stylish; if you choose one big light, make sure it's placed centrally over the table. If it's a long light, make sure it runs a good proportion of the length of the table and that the centre of the light starts in the middle of the table. If opting for multiple hanging pendants, make sure they are equal distance from each other so that they look symmetrical.

★ **ATMOSPHERE**

It doesn't have to take much to generate the perfect atmosphere around the dining table and doing so can also help to create memorable dining experiences. Taking into consideration the design and organisation tips above, it will then be a simple case of setting the tone by dimming your lighting, playing some chilled music and maybe even lighting a candle!

DINING ROOMS COME IN ALL SHAPES AND SIZES, BUT THE AIM OF THE GAME IS TO MAKE MEALTIMES AS MAGICAL AS POSSIBLE – THEY'RE A TIME TO CONNECT WITH LOVED ONES OR HAVE SOME CALM AT THE END OF THE DAY. FOCUS ON SMALL STYLE ADDITIONS WITH BIG IMPACT, FUNCTIONALITY, STORAGE AND MAKING THE VERY BEST OF THE SPACE YOU HAVE AVAILABLE!

the small dining room

If you don't have the space for a large dining table, consider an extendable table and extra folding chairs for when you have more guests than usual. Having a bench along one side of the table, instead of chairs, is also great for squeezing more people in and can be tucked away when not in use. Having a transparent table or chairs will help to create an illusion of more space. Adding a mirror near the table area will bounce light around the room.

If space is incredibly tight, minimise the furniture and consider only having out what is truly essential. Try a slimline console table that takes up minimal precious flooring and fit tall vertical shelving to store your special glasses, plates and dinnertime items.

Having a smaller space is something you can take advantage of, as it's an opportunity to design a beautiful, cosy and intimate space. If you love the look of dark, moody walls but think this isn't possible in a small dining room, this isn't the case! Try to keep your skirting and furniture light.

the large dining room

If you have a larger dining area, then take advantage of this space by having a beautiful, big dining table as your statement piece.

Having a large dining table also gives you the chance to have enough chairs to entertain and you can use these to bring in a pop of colour or texture to the room.

Choose a sideboard, bespoke cabinets or a unit to home items that need to be stored in this room. If you really envisage this as a social space, size permitting, you could even curate a bar area. Hire a carpenter to measure up what might work to fit the space perfectly or simply add a large drinks trolley.

Handy reminder: The Process

TO-DO CHECKLIST

- [ ] **Pull everything out** – empty every cupboard!
- [ ] **Detox** what is not longer serving the space
- [ ] **Categorise** and contain
- [ ] **Label**

WHAT YOU NEED CHECKLIST

- [ ] bin bags
- [ ] vacuum cleaner
- [ ] cleaning products
- [ ] storage boxes/containers
- [ ] label machine/labels

The Style Sisters guide to styling your . . .
dining table

We absolutely love styling our table place settings when we have guests. Special occasions and seasonal times of the year call for the table to be decorated and styled in different ways.

1. TABLECLOTH
Our classic look is to cover the table with a simple, neutral tablecloth as this instantly makes the table feel like you are at a posh restaurant and if there are any spillages or stains then they can be easily washed out.

2. PERFECT POSITIONING
Depending on the style of the table setting, you can place a charger plate, table mat or even a large slate tile underneath the plates to position the place settings. Place the cutlery in the correct position for dining, then add a wine glass along with a glass for water to finish this off perfectly.

3. NAPKINS
A cloth napkin placed on top of the plates, pulled in together with a napkin ring, ribbon or jute string, depending on your style of décor for the table, makes it feel like a special occasion. If you want to add names to the place settings, this can be done with luggage tags with your guests' names written in pretty handwriting. You can also add a touch of greenery, flower or sprig of herbs on top for that final special touch.

Now your table looks pretty, it's time to enjoy your dinner party and have a lovely time with your guests.

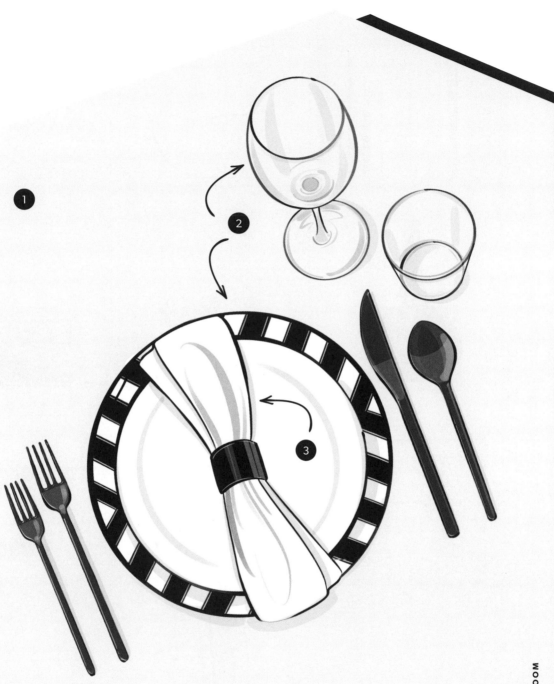

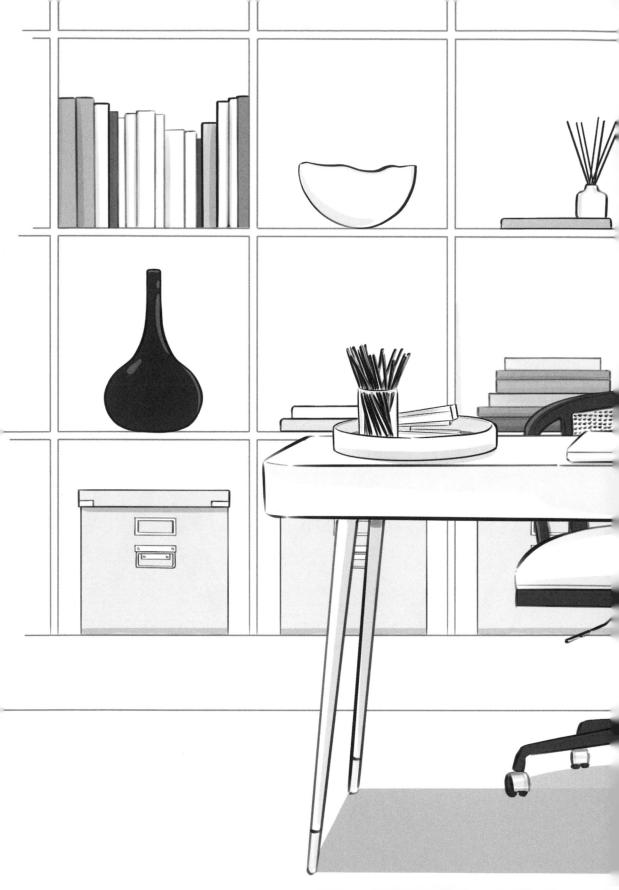

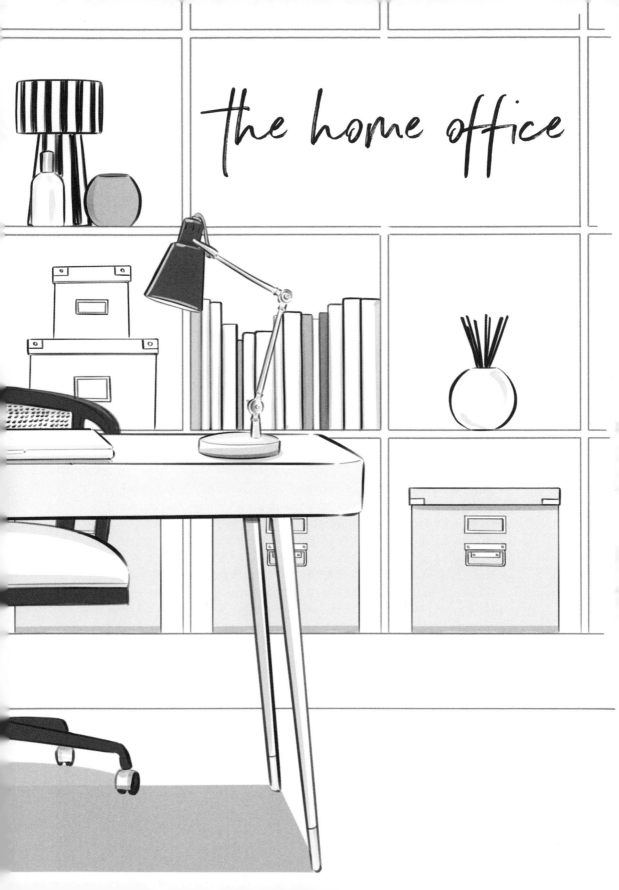

the home office

the home office

WORKING FROM HOME WILL BE A BREEZE

A lot of us are now working from home, if not full-time then at least a couple of days a week, and curating a productive and motivating space is essential for a good day's workand for boosting your wellbeing when it all gets too much. If you don't have a designated room for your home office, it's not a problem – we can help you create an organised office space anywhere around the house. Rolling out of bed and working from your sofa is probably not the best way to have a prouctive day, so structuring a zone or area to work from, such as your own work station, will help you feel more organised and ready for a stimulating day at the home office!

HOME OFFICE AREA

It doesn't take much to design a working zone in your home, it just depends on the space you have to work with. If you have a spare room that you have decided will become a home office this is a great idea. This can always be a temporary space and the room can revert back to being a guest room again in no time. If you already have furniture that can double up as a desk, such as a dressing table that is at the correct height to sit at comfortably, this can be used. However, if you don't have anywhere to sit, we suggest investing in a desk or a console table that is the correct height and has adequate space to sit at and work from. You need to be comfortable and in an environment that works for your work needs.

Another option is a foldaway table that can be stored easily so you can work from a sofa or comfy chair but have somewhere to put your laptop without having to balance it on your lap and risk injuring your back or neck. There are some really cool tables that fold away from the wall with artwork on the bottom, so they look like a piece of art, or even a blackboard, when folded. (These are also fun options for a kids' playroom.)

If you can, set up your workspace near a window or somewhere that has good ventilation and natural lighting as these are important for concentration and mood levels. Having plug sockets and power points nearby is essential to keep your laptop and phone going throughout the day.

We are all on a lot more Zoom and Teams meetings nowadays, so consider what your background is saying. Having a nice, tidy and clear background will appear more professional and won't distract all of your colleagues while on the call. It's all these little things that you need to take into consideration when setting up your work zone.

If you don't have the space for a desk, there are a few alternative solutions. Working from your kitchen table, kitchen island or living room table are obvious options and provide a desk-like surface and seating. If you can group your work items into a portable desk, you can set up in the morning and clear your 'desk' away in the evenings when the table needs to be used for eating or other purposes (see overleaf). If you have a dressing table, this can also double up as a desk in the same way.

Making sure you have a comfy and supportive chair is key when working from home. An office chair can look quite unsightly randomly placed around the home; if sat at one end of the dining table it can ruin the style of the room, so it works better behind an actual desk in an office room. But there are other chair options, for example bar stools that are adjustable in height are handy if you want to move your work station around the home. If you are using a dining chair for your desk chair, consider purchasing a back support. You can pick these up online for under £20 and they give your back a natural, curved support and releases pressure from sitting on a hard-backed chair all day.

top tip

A blackboard wall or acrylic calendar is a great idea for the office (or kitchen diner area) if you have a busy schedule with lots of meetings. These can look stylish and are practical to use and wipeable!

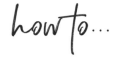

CREATE A PORTABLE DESK

If you don't have a permanent office space, purchase a little caddy with a handle to contain your work essentials that you can carry around your home to wherever you are setting up for the day.

In the caddy include items like pens, paper, notebooks, chargers, which can be stored alongside your laptop. Storing these things together stops them cluttering up other areas of your home and means you know exactly where all these work-related items are. Keeping them contained together also helps you to keep what you need for work streamlined and prevents you accumulating items that you don't need or use.

HOME OFFICE ROOM

If you have been working from your own home office for a while, then it is likely that, just as in other rooms, you will have built up clutter and the space will benefit from a good detox and organise. As always, please follow the steps we outlined in The Process on pages 36–9.

Essentials for an office include: pens, highlighters, Post-It notes, Sellotape, paperclips, Tipp-Ex, notepads, paper, stapler and staples... If you have items that you hardly ever use and they are taking up valuable space, it's time for them to go. Test all of your pens to make sure they still work as there's nothing worse than grabbing a pen to make notes and it's dried up!

The best way to store paperwork is in box files divided into categories that are relevant to you. Suggested categories include: household bills, bank statements and insurance details. Each piece of paper needs to be put into its correct subject file and then placed in the box file, then label the file with the category. It's then easy to file relevant paperwork as soon as you receive it and this helps to prevent it piling up. If you are lucky enough to have a designated room for your home office, you have a much wider choice of desks, chairs and other furniture. Your choice of desk is important,

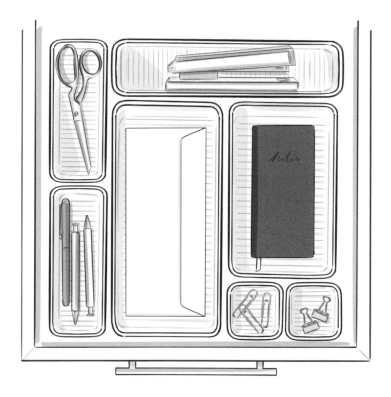

so consider how much storage it has. Does it have drawers, cupboards or a filing drawer for bills and paperwork? If it does, clever organisation in these drawers is a must; drawer dividers or containers in the drawers are useful for keeping everything nice and tidy. It is especially crucial for your desk, to make an investment to a piece of furniture that is actually functional, for your needs and the floor space.

top tip

Somewhere to store your pens and stationery is a top priority in an office – you don't want to be rummaging through a messy drawer to find a pen. Try storing them in a stylish pen pot or in a drawer divider which sections the drawer into compartments – this would be ideal in the top drawer of a desk. Stationery like staples, Sellotape and scissors should be contained together as they're essential items – think of them like a family who all need to live happily together – practicality makes for an easy life!

A lot of people have noticed health benefits from standing desks, and desks where the height can be adjusted are ideal for people who suffer with bad backs.

If you like the idea of having a stylish desk that is more like a console-style table or a glass desk, which we love, you need to make sure that you have space around the room for storage. A bookcase, sideboard or shelves are essential for a well-organised office and once you have the storage it's then all about the organisation inside!

top tip

A wooden or ottoman chest can double as seating and a filing unit for papers.

Floating shelves are handy for storing items and you can place storage boxes on them to hold all your office essentials. Try to make sure they are matching to keep the space looking stylish and co-ordinated. We love to use hard cardboard boxes in an office area – make sure you label each box so you know where everything is and this will keep you super organised.

If you are lacking surface space, it's a great idea to think vertically and make the best use of any available wall space. You can hang wire baskets on the walls to hold post, paperwork to do/file, or certain bits of stationery that you want to keep within easy reach.

Wire (or cable) tidies are a must in an office as you don't want a load of chargers and wires all getting tangled up together. You can also use cable ties to wrap up excess wires if they are too long.

A big bulbous printer/scanner can sometimes be a bit of an eyesore in a home office, but as it's often an essential, there are clever ways to conceal it, so it doesn't have to be on show. If you have a sideboard unit, check if the printer can fit on a shelf. If so, you can store it there and drill a hole in the back of the unit to allow the plug to fit through and hide the wire going into the plug point. A large storage box can also be used for the printer to sit in and it can then be removed when needed.

TOP TIPS for
a stylish home office

★ **INSPIRATIONAL ARTWORK**
We like to make our clients' home offices personal and stylish and adding artwork that inspires them and puts them in a good mood is a great place to start. Memorabilia, medals or trophies are also a popular items to showcase in a workspace. It's a room of work-related memories and these can also subconsciously promote feelings of success and inspire you to work more productively.

★ **COLOUR FOR CONCENTRATION**
The choice of colour in a home office is important – you don't want to paint the walls in a shade that is too vibrant or stimulating as it can become overwhelming after a while. Blue is often seen as an intellectual colour, so a nice rich blue would work well, and teamed up with white and brass accents it makes a stylish combo.

★ **THINK ABOUT LIGHTING**
Lighting in an office is another aspect to consider closely. Do you need a desk light as well as lamps, ceiling lights or wall lights? You want to be able to read any documents easily and so your workspace needs to be bright and well lit – you don't want to be falling asleep at your desk!

★ **ALWAYS ADD GREEN**
Adding greenery and fresh plants is a must in the Style Sisters' rule book, especially in an office. Plants help to promote the flow of oxygen around the room and bring life to the space as well as a lovely pop of colour. Add a succulent on your desk for a little pick-me-up, or treat yourself for working so hard with a pretty bunch of fresh flowers!

★ **FRAGRANCE FOR FOCUS**
Candles and diffusers are a wonderful addition to a work area. An uplifting scent will get your imagination going and awaken your senses, making you more alert and focused. Just remember to choose your scents carefully; you don't want a relaxing lavender candle in the office as you might get too relaxed and no work will get done!

'THANK YOU FOR HELPING ME DETOX MY WARDROBE LIKE NEVER BEFORE. EVERYONE NEEDS THESE LADIES IN THEIR LIVES.'

Lisa Snowdon

Handy reminder: The Process

TO-DO CHECKLIST

The following can be applied whether you are tackling an area at a time or completing the whole room at once!

- [ ] **Get everything out**
- [ ] **Check paperwork**, categorise and file
- [ ] **Make sure** you have a place for paperwork
- [ ] **Buy containers/divider**s for items in drawers
- [ ] **Buy storage solutions**, baskets or boxes to home items if they have nowhere to go
- [ ] **Purchase accessories** and display items for desk area

WHAT YOU NEED CHECKLIST

- [ ] bin bags
- [ ] vacuum cleaner
- [ ] cleaning products
- [ ] storage boxes/containers
- [ ] label machine/labels
- [ ] drawer dividers

The Style Sisters
guide to styling your . . .
desk

When it comes to styling your desk, you want it to be a calm and organised space. You don't want clutter building up that can cause distraction and may make you feel overwhelmed. Tidy home, tidy mind! This is a space you might be spending hours of your day in, so make sure it's streamlined and brings you much-needed boosts of visual joy amidst the daily stresses.

1. STORAGE
Decorative storage solutions are really helpful for keeping everything tidy and compact, but also stylish.

2. STATIONERY
Keep stationery contained in decorative pots – if you can get a matching or co-ordinated set it will make your desk space look super stylish.

3. TABLE LAMP
A lamp is a great addition to a desk and gives you an extra source of light if working late.

4. PLANTS
Plants add colour and life to a space. Adding a small succulent to your desk can help you feel uplifted and boost oxygen levels in the room, or a fresh vase of flowers brings the outdoors in and when stuck indoors all day will brighten your mood.

5. CHAIR
A comfy and supportive chair that adjusts to your height and has wheels is essential.

6. DESK
Choose a desk that is sturdy, durable and sleek and position it close to plug sockets.

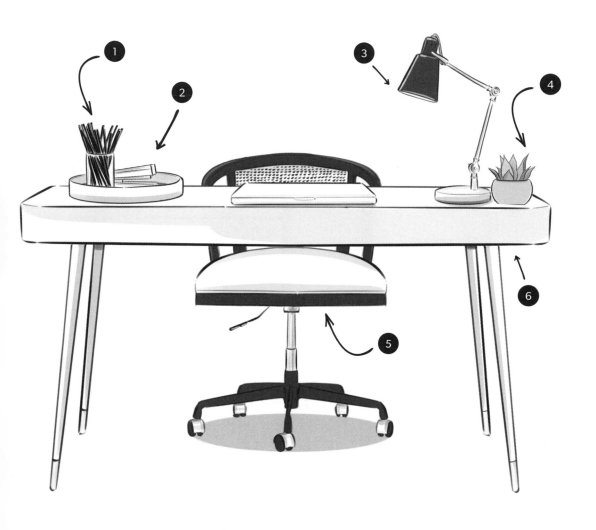

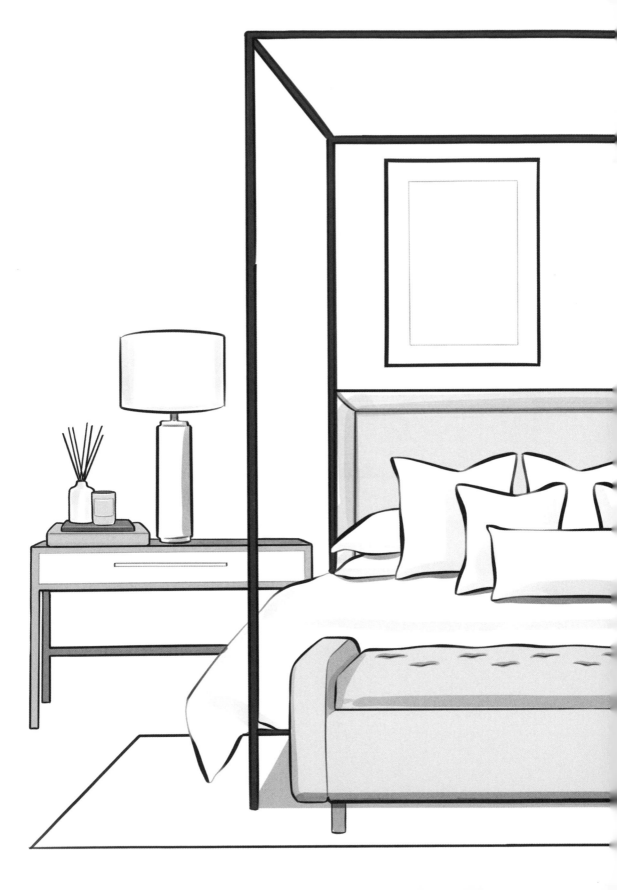

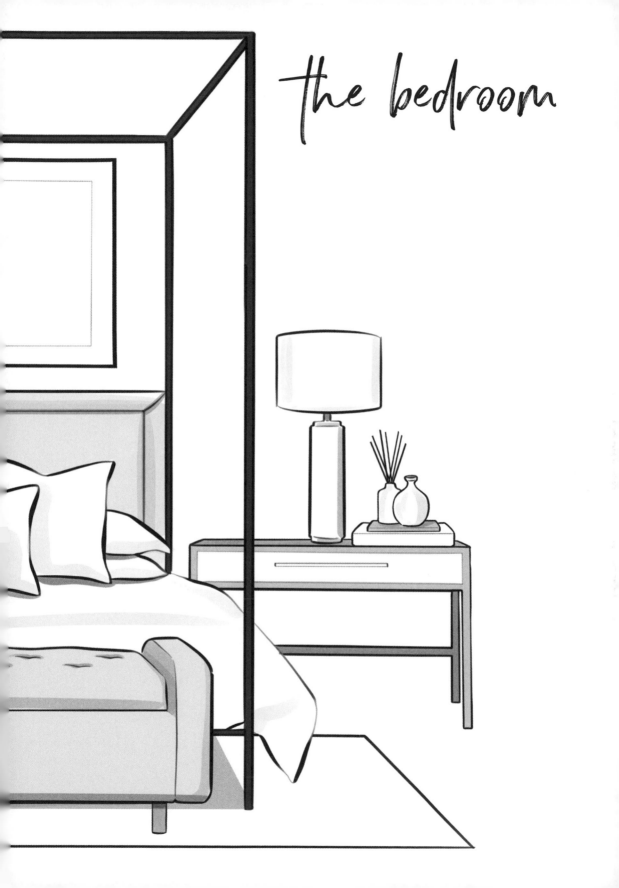

the bedroom

the bedroom

YOUR PERSONAL SANCTUARY

Your bedroom is not only where you begin each morning and get ready for the day ahead, but it is also the room where you go to rest and recharge in the evening. This is why we think your bedroom is one of the most important rooms in your home.

Having a beautiful, comfortable and cosy oasis where you can shut the door after a long day is key to enjoying your whole home. If your bedroom is a messy, disorganised space, it will stop you relaxing and will subconsciously be making you feel anxious, stressed and discontent, which isn't the right vibe at all.

It's common for the bedroom to become a bit of a dumping ground. Guests are coming round so you might pop a few items that are cluttering downstairs into your bedroom to hide them out of sight. Laundry piles up on the floor waiting to be put away. You may run out of space on your dressing table, so items make their way on to the bedside tables. All of a sudden, the room is a cluttered mess and can quickly become overwhelming. We've all had a 'floordrobe' at one point or another, or that chair that's covered in clothes.

In an ideal world your bedroom would consist of a bed, hardly any furniture and minimal electronics – essentially a really calm and neutral space to sleep. However, in the real world there is often lots of furniture and items to contend with and finding homes for these things can sometimes prove difficult.

This is why having a good detox is really important for the organisation of the room. Once you've decided what gets to stay, you can then assess the storage that's needed. We often find items that don't belong in a bedroom – shoved under beds, in the backs of wardrobes or cupboards – and this isn't good for your state of mind or the state of the room.

We know it sounds daunting, but it really is a case of getting everything out and creating piles of keep, give, sell, or get rid. Follow our steps in The Process on pages 36–9. With every item that has been hidden in a drawer or the back of a cupboard, be honest with yourself – when was the last time you used it or have even seen it? It's obviously been hiding for a reason! You need to work out what items you need, use and want.

The bedroom should be homing items and products that you need to go to sleep, a wardrobe if you don't have a separate dressing area, a dressing table or somewhere to sit and get ready, and a chest of drawers or storage for items like underwear and pyjamas. Items like work papers, computers, unread books and magazines, and even exercise bikes, are all stopping you from enjoying the purpose of your bedroom. Remember this is the one room in the house where you NEED to be able to switch off and unwind. Sleep is so important for your well-being and not having the right setting will most definitely have a huge impact on the quality of sleep you will have.

Consider other areas of the home where items can live. Really think about the layout of your home and where you would ideally love everything to be. Compromises may need to be made depending on the space you have, but planning where these items would ideally live is a good place to start. Do you have any items that you are doubling up on? Products you no longer need or use? When was the last time you sorted through your make-up and discarded any dried up nail polishes? When did you last check the expiry dates on your products? Often, without realising it, you can be holding on to items that are taking up valuable space and it's time for an overhaul!

PRACTICAL FURNITURE

Utilising every possible area for storage if you are tight on space is crucial in smaller rooms, especially a bedroom, because you don't want them to feel overcrowded and cluttered with furniture. So, you have to be clever with what pieces you purchase and use.

Storage beds are an amazing option; you get two practical uses out of one item – somewhere to sleep and somewhere to store. You can either get a bed with storage drawers or one that lifts up from the mattress, so you get the area under the bed for storage. We have used these spaces in clients' homes for shoes, bed linen, memory boxes (see page 28), electronics and sports clothing such as ski suits. Make sure these items are not ones you use daily, as lifting your bed every day can become a bit of a mission!

If you have space at the end of your bed for an ottoman footstool, you can purchase hollow ones with a lift-up top if you need extra storage for items without a home. You could add a slimline version in the same place or go for a smaller round one to sit nicely in the corner. If you have a chair in your bedroom, you could perhaps opt for an ottoman instead, so you gain extra storage while still having somewhere to sit.

The pieces of furniture you choose for your bedroom need to be practical with lots of drawer space – large, deep drawers are ideal if you are short on room. It's better to have one larger unit with decent-sized drawers than a few pieces of furniture with tiny drawers you can hardly fit anything in taking up more room and making the space feel cluttered. We have never had a client say they have too much storage space, so the more you have the better – always!

Bedside tables are important; we've found over the years working with clients and from our own personal experience that they are somewhere where you often need to store a lot of random bits and bobs. They might home a lamp if you don't have pendant or wall lights, a pillow spray, a sleep mask, night creams, lip balm, a Kindle or book, notebook and pen, chargers, torch (in case of a power cut, it's a practical item to have), candle… the list goes on. You don't want all these items randomly scattered on top of the unit, so by having a good-sized drawer you can section it into different compartments and then organise the items so that they can be easily found.

By all means keep a few decorative items on display, like a candle and pillow spray, but the idea is for the bedside unit to be clutter-free neat, to encourage you to totally let go before you drift off.

PUT IT AWAY

If your wardrobe is in your bedroom, make sure clothing and shoes go back into their designated space and don't end up thrown on to the floor or flung over a chair – this is not chilled out bedroom vibes! The best way to avoid this happening is every item having a home. Mess builds over time up when you don't know where to put something or you don't have enough space. This is why having a regular detox can prevent this from happening.

If you have space above the wardrobe for storage baskets this is ideal. Make sure you get boxes that match the interior of the bedroom or opt for a similar colour to the wardrobe, so it looks aesthetically pleasing to the eye.

LOVELY LINENS

If you are storing bed linens, bed sheets and pillowcases in your bedroom, make sure you have matching sets and check them all over to make sure they all fit the bed and are still in good condition. We like to fold duvets up with their matching pillowcases and then take one of the cases and place the set inside the case, so when you pick up the case it's like a little parcel of the bed linen set. This can then be stored on a shelf, in an ottoman or in a large drawer (or in an airing cupboard if not storing in the bedroom).

top tip

Completing a simple task like making your bed every morning will make you feel more organised and content. Plus, your bedroom will look a million times better than if the pillows and cushions are all thrown over the floor and the duvet is in a heap on the bed. Try to start the day in a positive and structured way and make making your bed a part of your wake-up routine!

DRESSING TABLE DOS

If your dressing table is in your bedroom and this is where you get ready every day, having the drawers sectioned into categories is a must!

Depending on the size of the drawers, how many products you have and what needs to be stored here, we ideally like to organise the drawers as if you are working on your face. If you have a classic dressing table with drawers either side of where you sit, we suggest working from the top left as the face drawer: face creams, serums, foundations and concealers; the drawer below that will be another face drawer with bronzer, powders and blusher/highlighters: the drawers to the right will be an eye drawer for eyeliners, mascaras, brows and eyeshadows: and below that a lip drawer for lip glosses, lipsticks and lip liners. This concept and layout can also apply if you have all your items in one drawer.

Depending on how big the drawers are, you might be able to fit some stackable drawer divider trays in there and section items into each divider, so separating your lip drawer into lip glosses, lipsticks and lip liners for example. If your drawers aren't large enough for divider trays, extendable drawer dividers are a great option as you can adjust the size of the section you need in the drawer. Alternatively, you can use cardboard boxes from packaging to make your own dividers.

Having a drawer for your haircare items is always really handy too. These are items that are often needed and can sometimes be left without a home. Items such as hairbrushes, hairbands and clips, plus a hairdryer and straighteners, are ones you're likely to use often, so having a drawer or decorative basket for these is helpful. Things like hair masks and curlers are items you're probably not using all the time, so you can consider new homes for these if space is an issue.

A pretty tray placed on the top of the dressing table makes a stylish and practical way of displaying and storing your perfume bottles and decorative pieces.

Client Stories

If you would love a dressing table in your bedroom but you don't have the space, think outside the box! We had a lovely client who was desperate for a dressing table in her bedroom, but the room was an odd shape and there simply wasn't the space for a traditional one. However, we didn't want to be defeated and were determined to try to find a way to give her the space she desired. We decided to go for a freestanding mirror that had a shelf at the bottom, paired with a dressing table stool. We then placed a decorative shelf on the wall next to the mirror and displayed the client's perfumes and other bits and bobs on it. This hack took up minimal space but allowed our client to have the space she desired, just not exactly how she had initially envisioned it. We were all over the moon with how it turned out and it looked really beautiful. There is always a way to achieve the space you desire – within reason – you just sometimes have to think outside the box and be willing to compromise on your initial vision.

TOP TIPS for a stylish bedroom

★ **BED REST**

There are so many bed styles to choose from – upholstered, metal, four-poster or wooden – and it's an important feature of the room and can set the tone for this space. Think about the design element and how you want this room to look when deciding on the style of bed you buy, but don't forget that comfort is just as important as style. You are sleeping in your bed every night, so its main purpose is to help you feel as rested and rejuvenated as possible.

The type of mattress you have is really important for getting a good night's sleep. Everyone has a personal preference as to whether they prefer a hard, soft or memory foam mattress… it can be a minefield of choices! How firm your mattress is will affect how well you sleep. The type of firmness you need will depend on your sleeping position, height and weight. Below is a guide to what level of firmness is best depending on what type of sleeper you are:

Soft: Side sleepers or those who change positions during the night are best suited to soft mattresses. This is because the way you sleep already relieves pressure from your spine so you want your mattress to mould to your body's natural position.

Medium soft: This is ideal for those who change their sleeping position during the night, as it will still mould to your body position but provide a little more support.

Medium firm: This is best for people who sleep on their back as you require extra lower-back support, which this type of firmness offers.

Firm: This type of mattress is ideal for those who sleep on their front, are over 15 stone or suffer from back pain because it will keep your back in a relatively comfortable and stable position without allowing you to sink into the mattress as you sleep, which can cause lower back pain.

You also need to think about size – you don't want to swamp the room with a super-king-size bed if you only have a small space. You might want to try a large double or king and have a little more floor space around the bed, so you don't have to perform some crazy acrobatics to get into bed every night!

When choosing bedding for your bed, opt for top-quality bed sheets with a high thread count as it will make your bed feel that little bit more luxurious, plus they will last longer. There are a variety of different fabrics you can choose from – smooth satin, soft linen and cotton – so go for what you prefer. With bedding, opt for quality over quantity if you can.

★ CALM COLOUR

The choice of colour in your bedroom is also important as you want it to be a calm and chilled space. Bright, vibrant colours that keep you alert and active are not a wise choice in a bedroom, so stay away from these and also from dark reds and blacks as they can be too heavy and oppressive in a space where you should be resting (see page 196 for more guidance on choosing colours and the best places to use them).

We love to style our clients' bedrooms with neutral colours. Popular shades are off-white, greige and taupe, and then we then add lots of textures and tones in the same colour palette to the room using accessories and soft textiles to help the space feel calm, luxurious and interesting. The bedroom is a great place to add a little texture and colour to the room with wallpaper. If you choose a wallpaper with a pattern, the golden rule is to not use any more than three patterns, for example a herringbone, stripe and geometric. Be careful about adding other patterns to the room. This rule is especially important when deciding on the cushions to place on the bed.

★ LOW LIGHTING

We have touched on the spotlight situation in the Dining Room chapter (see page 100) and the bedroom is definitely somewhere where spotlights should be forbidden. They cast shadows on your face if you have a dressing table in the room, so you want dimmable lighting if you do have spotlights, or if you have a statement pendant light a dimmer will work well too.

We like to introduce a moodier setting in a bedroom by using lamps with warm bulbs for a softer, sexier vibe. Hanging pendant lights next to the bed are a lovely feature and can give a hotel room look that so many of our clients are after, to curate that space of escapism.

★ **CONSIDER YOUR WINDOW TREATMENTS**

Window treatments are a key factor in the bedroom. Some people need complete darkness to get to sleep while others prefer to have sheer curtains to wake them up when the sun rises – it's all personal preference. We love to make the windows a feature so choosing which blinds or curtains to use is an important decision.

If you want light-coloured curtains (we love using light fabrics to dress bedroom windows) but want to get a good night's sleep with not much light coming through, you can overcome this by getting them blacked out or having a thicker lining sewn in if you are having them made. This will make them thicker and they will also hang nicely.

If you have Roman blinds in the bedroom, we also love to include a sheer blind that sits underneath. This adds an extra layer of privacy but doesn't stop or block the natural light coming through.

If shutters or wooden blinds are more your style, these work just as well in the bedroom as in the rest of the home.

★ **COSY CARPET**

Carpet is lovely in the bedroom as it adds warmth and comfort under your feet and a feeling of luxury. If you have hard flooring, consider getting a nice large rug that will go under the bed and will cover both sides so when you get up in the morning you can feel the fabric under your feet. The sizing of the rug is key for it to look right. If you don't want to splurge out on a large rug, another great way of adding cosiness is getting smaller rugs or runners that can be placed either side of the bed. These will keep your feet nice and warm when getting out of bed in the morning and also add that extra bit of texture to the room. We love to use sheepskin, faux fur or hides or jute rugs in the bedroom. Don't forget you can also layer rugs to add an extra bit of interest.

★ **FAVOURITE PHOTOS**

Adding family photos or pictures that you love and that inspire you is a lovely touch in the bedroom. After all, this is the place where you fall asleep, so seeing these images just before you drift off and as soon as you wake up inspires a nice feeling and conjures positive memories to start and end the day with. Alternatively, you can add artwork to the walls for a pop of colour and style.

★ PERFECT PLANTS

Plants look great in a bedroom and will lift your mood and add a feel-good vibe. Try not to choose anything too large as this can be overpowering in the room. Stick with smaller choices like succulents and potted plants that can fit on a chest of drawers or bedside table. (See page 206 for our favourite houseplants.)

★ RELAXING FRAGRANCE

Fragrance is an essential aspect of a bedroom and a way to elevate it to a calm and content space. Try to use relaxing scents that will help with a good night's sleep; lavender is a popular go-to for winding down and reducing anxiety levels. If you don't want candles in the bedroom, try an oil diffuser or a lavender mist or sleep spray to spritz on to your pillows to aid a good night's sleep.

top tip

Getting the temperature right in the bedroom is key to a good night's sleep. Set the thermostat a little lower than the rest of the house and/or make sure any radiators are turned to a lower setting than other rooms. Open a window slightly so that a soft breeze can enter the room and keep the fresh air circulating.

★ GET COSY

For a spa-like experience in your own home, invest in a high-quality cotton dressing robe and plush slippers so you can relax and chill out while getting ready for bed. Being cosy and warm will make you feel more content and relaxed before a peaceful night's sleep. The same rule goes for including a beautiful selection of comfortable and comforting soft furnishings.

the small bedroom

If your bedroom is on the smaller side, you have to be clever with how you use the space.

A bed that works well in the room and still gives you enough space to move around is crucial. If you need to home your clothes and shoes in the bedroom, fitted wardrobes are a great investment as they will use every bit of available space in a more practical way than freestanding wardrobes. Ottoman storage beds are great way to utilise what would have been unused space. By choosing floor-to-ceiling designs you will also maximise your space and storage. If you need a chest of drawers for storage, make sure it is a good size for the room. Double-check the drawer size and depth as it is better to have fewer larger drawers than more drawers with less space in them.

If you need somewhere to sit and do your hair and make-up but the room is too small for a dressing table, a floating dressing table attached to the wall with a small stool to sit on is a practical way of using less space but still giving you an area where you can sit and get ready (see Client Stories, page 125).

the large bedroom

If you have a large bedroom, you can really go to town on a large feature bed and dressing tables with storage as you have space to play with.

If you have a large flat wall where the bed will be coming from, having a headboard wall that's either mirrored, fabric or padded is an interesting feature in a larger bedroom.

If you need clothes storage, fitted wardrobes are a great investment as you can have just one wall kitted out with wardrobe space, hanging clothes rails and drawers, which then frees up space to perhaps have a lovely accent chair and side table or dressing table, so the room then becomes more hotel chic than furniture store.

Handy reminder: The Process

TO-DO CHECKLIST

The following can be applied whether you are tackling one area at a time or completing the whole room at once:

- [ ] **Empty** every cupboard and drawer
- [ ] **Work out what can be kept**, moved to another room, donated or thrown
- [ ] **Check expiry dates** on make-up and chuck if out of date or it has been open for a while
- [ ] **Remove** items from the room that don't belong in a bedroom
- [ ] **Buy storage solutions**, baskets or boxes to home items with nowhere to go
- [ ] **Add** a calming scent

WHAT YOU NEED CHECKLIST

- [ ] bin bags
- [ ] vacuum cleaner
- [ ] cleaning products
- [ ] storage boxes/containers
- [ ] label machine/labels
- [ ] drawer dividers
- [ ] vacuum pack bags

The Style Sisters
guide to styling your . . .
bed

Cushions on the bed are a perfect way to add colour and texture to the bedroom. We recommend two sleeping pillows followed by a large 60 x 60cm continental cushion in front of the sleeping pillows and then by a display of cushions – six at the most. You want the bed to look cosy, luxe and inviting but you don't want to be spending ages dismantling the cushions before you get into bed every night!

Work with the colour scheme of the room – if you want to add an accent colour, just remember to keep all the colours in sync with each other. If you want to add pattern, the rule of three applies here (see page 200), and make sure all patterns use the same colour palette. A good solid-colour cushion works well, followed with a patterned or striped cushion and you can also add different textures with cushions too.

This will make the bed look more interesting and will add style to the room. Don't be afraid to go big with your cushions – small little pillows on the bed will look lost and won't achieve the grand impact you want.

Remember, if you purchase cushions and they already have the cushion inners inside and they are a flat microfibre, you can replace them with a feather filled inners. These will instantly be plumper and sit nicely on the bed.

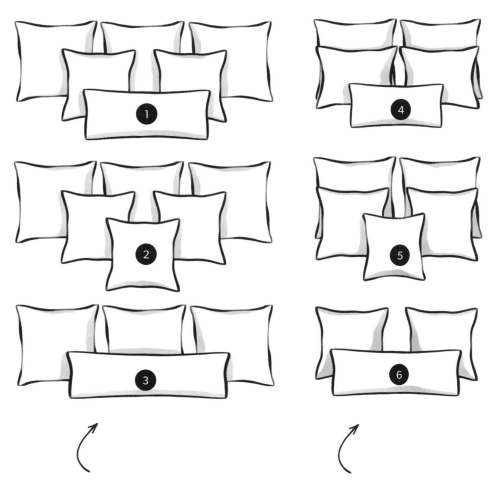

LARGER BEDS

The cushion arrangement on 1, 2 and 3 are for larger beds like king and super king.

SMALLER BEDS

The cushion arrangement on 4, 5 and 6 are for smaller beds like singles and doubles.

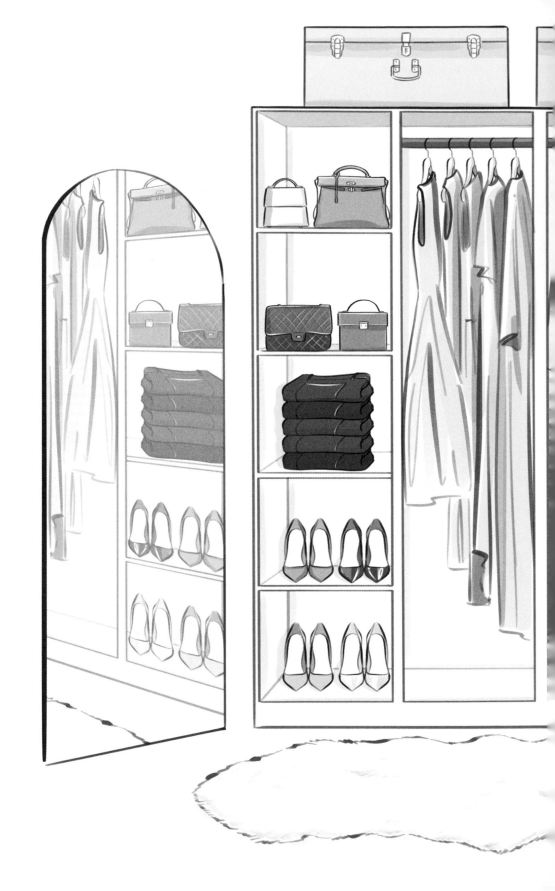

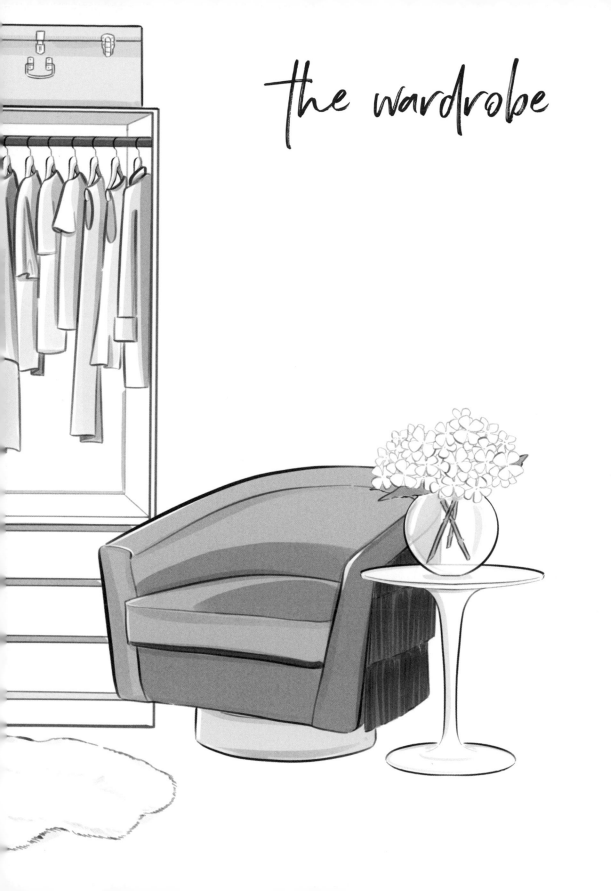

the wardrobe

the wardrobe

LOVE WHAT YOU WEAR, WEAR WHAT YOU LOVE

Whether you consider yourself into fashion or not, clothes are a necessity and can be a powerful form of self-expression. When you feel good in what you're wearing it automatically puts you in a better mood. How many times have you been wearing an outfit which just doesn't make you feel good and it's affected your confidence? Clothes are a way to showcase your style and tastes as well as convey how you are feeling.

We've both lost count of the number of times we've pulled on some comfy clothes because we're not in a happy state of mind or have reached for an item that we know will ensure we're feel on top of the world. There is no denying that we all have emotional attachments to clothes.

We go to our wardrobe several times a day and, let's face it, we couldn't leave the house without doing so. (Well, you could, and if you want to, we support you, but you may get cold in the winter!) So, your wardrobe should be a place that inspires you, not somewhere that stresses you out first thing in the morning. You may not even realise the subconscious effect a messy and disorganised wardrobe is having on your mood until you've organised it and witnessed the amazing benefits of a good wardrobe detox.

top tip

A great way to figure out what you're wearing and what you're not is to turn all the hangers in one direction and when you wear an item hang the hanger the opposite way. This way in 6 months time you will visually be able to see what you have worn and what you haven't, helping you in your next detox process.

THE DETOX

We recommend you detox your wardrobe at least once or twice a year, ideally when the season changes. Your wardrobe should be filled with clothes you love and that you actually want to wear. It should not be a place to store items you know you're never going to wear but are perhaps holding on to for one of many different reasons. Like a top you bought for a night out a few years ago, which you've worn once and have no real desire to wear again, but because you liked it then or you spent a small fortune on it, you're finding it hard to say goodbye. Detoxing your wardrobe requires you to be in the right head space; you need to be willing to be really honest with yourself about whether you're actually going to wear something again or whether you're keeping it for another reason. Maybe it's sentimental, like the outfit you were wearing when you met your partner, but whatever the reason, we will help you get to the bottom of it and place it in its rightful home, whether that's in a memory box (see page 28) or donating it to a friend's wardrobe. It doesn't matter how big your wardrobe is, the same rules apply. If you're not going to wear it, it needs to go!

To start, you want to make sure you get everything out. No drawer should be left unturned! Follow the steps we laid out for you in The Process on pages 36–9. Get absolutely everything out and create your four piles: keep, give, sell, get rid. Having somewhere to place your items helps you mentally when pulling clothes out of the wardrobe as it can often feel overwhelming to have to decide what to do with them. Taking items out of your wardrobe that you know you're never going to wear again frees up valuable space for items that you love and do wear regularly. You can place any special pieces of clothing in a memory box (see page 28), or you could even get creative and make something with them. It could be a blanket made from all of the items stitched together or a special piece of clothing can be placed in a frame to create a unique piece of artwork.

If you're unsure about something, try it on! We have lost count of the number of times our clients have not been sure about something, or they have loved it but not actually worn it in years. We always recommend that they try it on to help them make their decision. More often than not the item no longer fits, or they don't like how it looks any more, which makes the decision for them.

This is also where asking a trusted friend or family member can be really helpful. If you're not sure about something, ask someone whose opinion you value, or you could even take a photo of yourself in an outfit so you can see it from a different angle or send to a friend for their thoughts.

If you try something on and you like it, ask yourself how and where you would wear it. Do you need to purchase something to wear with it? Be realistic with yourself – there are only seven days in a week. Take into consideration whether you wear a uniform to work or what you spend most of your days wearing. Do you have to dress smartly for an office? Do you need a few formal outfits for meetings but can wear what you like the rest of the time? Are you ever going to get the chance to wear everything in your wardrobe? Probably not! So, if you're unsure about something, we're almost certain you won't wear it. You will always pick something you like more over an item that you're so-so on. Having lots of options is great if you love and want to wear all of them, but including clothes you know you won't wear just makes getting dressed harder! It is so much better to have quality over quantity. Less is sometimes more.

SHOP YOUR WARDROBE AND MAKE SPACE

Having a detox allows you to shop your wardrobe and rediscover items you had forgotten about. We often hear clients saying, 'I love this, and I'd forgotten I even had it!'. Creating a calm and organised wardrobe will allow you to see all your clothes so that you don't forget what you have.

If space is an issue, then a detox isn't the only thing you can do. Consider using vacuum-pack bags to store certain items you may not be wearing right now and think about creating a seasonal wardrobe. This is something we often recommend to our clients. There isn't much point looking at your winter knits on a hot summer's day! It makes so much more sense to only have your summer wardrobe hanging up in summer and the same goes for winter. You can store out-of-season items in vacuum-pack bags in decorative storage baskets on top of the wardrobe or even in suitcases which would otherwise be dead space. Get savvy about where you can store items and don't be afraid to think outside the box. It only has to make sense to you. If you're short on space, use under-the-bed storage wisely and also utilise wall space. You can use shelving to display your shoes. Consider the back of wardrobe doors for accessories and the back of doors for shoe shelves, which can be purchased inexpensively and allow you to store a minimum of 12 pairs of shoes!

HOW SHOULD I ORGANISE MY WARDROBE?

Look at your everyday living habits and decide what you need from your wardrobe. If you have lots of shoes, then your wardrobe needs to allow for this so they are not an afterthought. Do you go to the gym a lot? If so, exercise attire should take prime space over dressy outfits. Your wardrobe needs to suit you and your lifestyle, and having it organised in a way that serves you makes life so much easier.

One of our celebrity clients Vogue Williams is an active gym-goer (we would both like some of her motivation please!) but her wardrobe was not in sync with her lifestyle. She had gym clothes in various wardrobes and it just didn't work. We quickly decided after seeing the space that it made total sense to dedicate a whole area to her gym clothes and trainers, so they were all in one place. This allowed her to not only see everything but made getting dressed easier and quicker too.

This is why we always say: assess your space. Sometimes your wardrobe has become a place you put things without thinking about where they are going. You may have had a lifestyle change since your last wardrobe sort out and so you're battling for space for clothes you don't need any more. You may have changed jobs and gone from working in an office to becoming a gym instructor or started working freelance from home. You now have no need for the formal wear still taking up space in your wardrobe.

Detoxing and grouping similar items together hugely benefits the way your wardrobe works for you. It allows you to keep on top of what you have as opposed to buying more of the same thing because you can't see what you have and have forgotten what you own! We recommend organising your clothes by category and then colour-coordinating within that category. Keep jeans, knitwear, tops, work wear and dresses together, and then colour-coordinate within each of these categories. This allows you to find exactly what you need when you need it and also helps you make smarter buying decisions. If you can see that you have 15 white T-shirts whereas before you could never find one, it will stop you buying more!

Often when we are helping clients, we will suggest outfit ideas using certain pieces that they wouldn't have thought about pairing together. We can all sometimes get caught up in repetitive habits of how we wear things and can't see past them. Having your wardrobe organised so that you can see all your clothes will give you far more outfit inspiration.

SHOULD I KEEP IT?

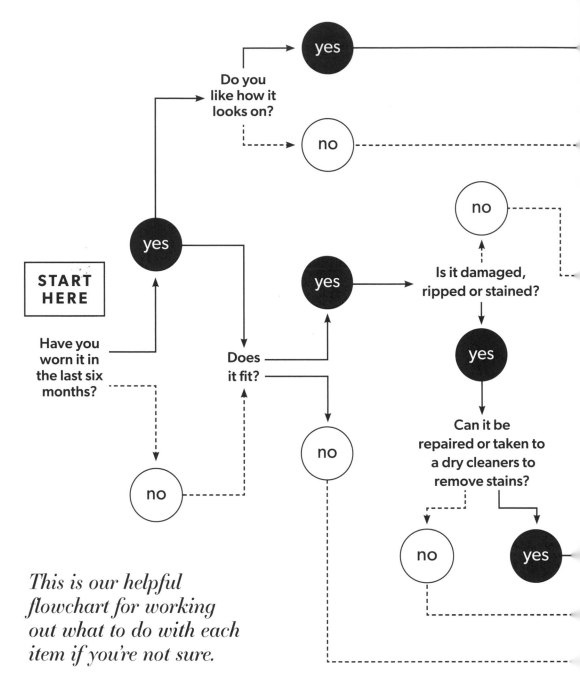

Do you like how it looks on?

yes

no

Is it damaged, ripped or stained?

no

yes

yes

Can it be repaired or taken to a dry cleaners to remove stains?

no

yes

yes

START HERE

Have you worn it in the last six months?

Does it fit?

yes

no

no

This is our helpful flowchart for working out what to do with each item if you're not sure.

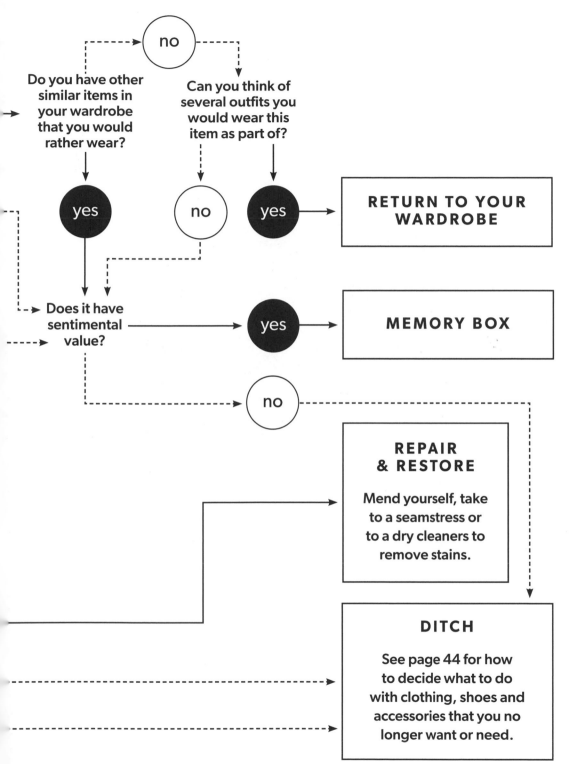

no

Do you have other similar items in your wardrobe that you would rather wear?

Can you think of several outfits you would wear this item as part of?

yes

no

yes

RETURN TO YOUR WARDROBE

Does it have sentimental value?

yes

MEMORY BOX

no

REPAIR & RESTORE

Mend yourself, take to a seamstress or to a dry cleaners to remove stains.

DITCH

See page 44 for how to decide what to do with clothing, shoes and accessories that you no longer want or need.

THE WARDROBE

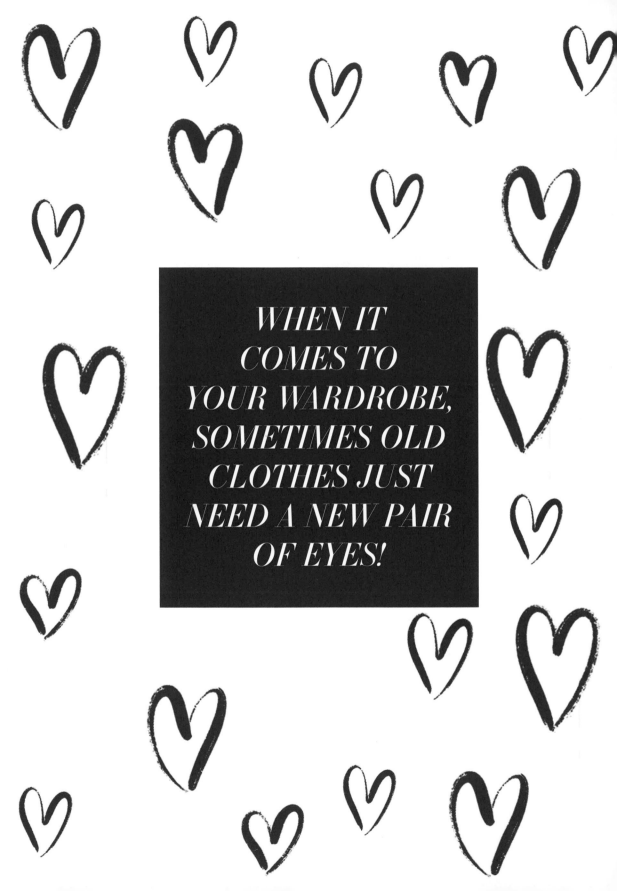

WHEN IT COMES TO YOUR WARDROBE, SOMETIMES OLD CLOTHES JUST NEED A NEW PAIR OF EYES!

KNITWEAR

We often are asked about how to store knitwear. We love to fold chunkier knits onto shelves as they are heavier, however we have also hung them too. We prefer to hang finer knits but it is all down to personal choice. Use special knitwear hangers to avoid your knitwear getting ruined from hanging.

ACCESSORIES

When it comes to putting away items like hats, scarves and belts, many people often don't know the best way to store or display them. Accessories are frequently overlooked and end up being stuffed in wherever they fit (or don't!) as an afterthought. This doesn't have to be the case though. Accessories can make an outfit and they should be stored so that you can easily see them and they're still serving a purpose in your life.

Our preferred way to tidy away accessories is to store them in drawers using drawer dividers. By dividing your drawer(s) into sections with dividers, you create more space than you would have without them. You can designate a section to each category of accessories. Fold and roll scarves so that they can be placed together in one section – they should each look like a little parcel when you're done. These can then be stored lined up, allowing you to see everything you have. Using a slimline drawer divider, you can also roll your belts and then place them one after the other in the divider, with the buckles facing up so you can see each style easily. Remember to colour-coordinate all items in the same way as you would your clothes.

You have now turned one drawer that may just have had a jumbled mass of scarves and belts stuffed in, into an organised accessories haven where you can see everything. You can use the other divided sections for items like your hats or gloves or any other accessories you want stored here. Remember, it only needs to make sense to you and for your lifestyle. The aim is for everything to have a home while allowing you to see it all. This way nothing gets forgotten about!

If drawer space isn't something you have, then consider decorative storage baskets and stick to the same principles as above. Scarves can also be kept on hooks or draped over hangers depending on what you prefer and the space you're working with.

SHOES

We get asked about shoes A LOT! From tips to storing them if space is an issue, to whether they should be kept in their boxes or not. Truthfully, there is no right or wrong answer, but make sure the organisation is space-saving and functional. We prefer to take shoes out of their boxes, providing they have a home and won't be thrown into a cupboard amongst a mass of other shoes (*sweating face emoji*). This way you actually get to see them and you're more likely to wear them. We have found our clients often end up forgetting about shoes if they are hidden away in boxes (the shoes have told us this makes them sad, and no-one wants sad shoes), so where it is possible, we always like to store them in a highly visible and clear way.

If, like both our partners, you can't cope with the idea of your shoes not being stored in their original boxes and won't be persuaded otherwise, then we have a few tips that will help you keep everything looking organised but also ensure you don't forget what you have!

★   Opt for or create a cupboard with shelves. This way you can stack the boxes and everything still looks neat.

★   Try putting the boxes along the top of your wardrobe if space is an issue or even storing them neatly under the bed with the label showing the style of shoe on the box on display.

★   If the number of boxes you have outweighs your space, think about whether you have a cupboard in the house that you could kit out with shelving to turn it into a shoe cupboard.

★   Take Polaroid pictures of the shoes and stick them on the front of the boxes so you have a visual reminder of what is inside.

★   Group shoeboxes together in categories, the same way you would if they were out on show, so for example, keep trainer boxes together.

★   You can purchase clear shoeboxes from sites like eBay and Amazon so you can see what shoes are in them without having to even open the box. Another benefit is that they are all matching, so you can have them on display if you need/want and it will still look aesthetically pleasing.

Client Stories

We had one client who had hundreds of pairs of shoes still in their boxes on a shelf. She could never see what she had and therefore, never wore any of them not immediately in view. We talked her through the benefits of having her shoes out of the boxes and she decided she wanted to try it. Once we had the go-ahead, Charlotte was like a kid at Christmas taking the boxes off the shelves and unpacking the shoes! When we had put the shoes away, not only did the shoe wall look so much better, but our client could now see everything she had with ease!

SELECT YOUR SHOE STORAGE

★ You can get clever under-the-bed storage bags that zip up and are divided into shoe sections. The top of the bag is clear so you can pull the bag out from under the bed and see what's inside easily.

★ Try over-the-door shoe hangers. These can be hung on the back of your bedroom door or a storage cupboard and, depending on the version you purchase, can hold 12–35 pairs of shoes.

★ There are so many amazing shoe rack options available and they can be bought fairly cheaply. These are a simple solution if you want to store your shoes out of the boxes but want them neatly on display. You can get tall ones that hold up to 40 pairs of shoes or extendable ones that can sit inside your wardrobe and expand to fit the width of the space.

★ Just as you can have a seasonal clothes wardrobe, the same applies for your shoes. Having only seasonally-appropriate shoes out at any one time – flip-flops and sandals in the summer, chunky boots in the winter – can free up some much-needed space.

When putting your shoes away, place them on the shelf with one facing forwards and one facing backwards and then alternate like this with all your shoes. This will maximise space, allowing you to get more shoes on the shelf.

BAGS

Bags are like shoes – they are good investments but can take up a lot of space and often leave people feeling frustrated with how to store them. We have a few tips and tricks to help you store your bags while still allowing you to see them!

Our preferred way of keeping bags stylishly organised is to display them on shelves. You tend to not use different bags as often as you might other items in your wardrobe, so they can be stored higher up. Remember, as long as you can still see them, they won't get forgotten about. We usually opt for the shelves at the top of the wardrobe or sit them along the top of the wardrobe itself. Remember to group your bags into colours for a beautiful, organised-looking finish. You can also keep larger bags and smaller bags together if desired; there is no right or wrong – like we always say, it's about what works for you! No matter what type of item you may be dealing with around the home, as long as items in the same category are kept together, you will always know where everything is and won't forget what you have.

Below are a few tips and tricks to consider when displaying your bags and ways you can save space:

★ Try using bag dividers if you're having trouble keeping your bags standing up. Or you can fill bags with newspaper stuffed into a carrier bag so that it's easy to take in and out when you want to use a bag. This stops them being floppy and helps make them easier to display.

★ Separate larger bags from smaller clutch bags if shelf space is an issue. You can store clutch bags in a drawer and larger bags on a shelf. If you're really tight on space, you can place clutch bags inside larger bags.

★ Consider placing hooks on walls to hang bags from. This totally depends on the space you have to work with. We would recommend this more in a dressing room/walk-in wardrobe (see page 153) than a bedroom with a wardrobe in. You can also place hooks on the inside of a wardrobe door.

★ Have you got an area you could place some floating shelves to store bags on? Remember to go for a deeper shelf so that the bags fit.

JEWELLERY

There are some amazing options available for storing your jewellery. When it comes to displaying and keeping it untangled, neat and organised, sectioning off the subcategories is a good starting point i.e. everyday bits, special earrings, bracelets, bigger statement pieces. Below are some ideas to consider – use the ones that you feel will work best for you and your space.

★   You can't beat a good old jewellery box! There are so many beautiful ones available and it should be easy to find one that matches the style of the space it will be placed in. We love stackable jewellery boxes. They take up less space and you can add to your collection without worrying about where pieces will be stored as you can always purchase another layer when it's needed.

★   Stick small hooks on the inside of your wardrobe door to display your necklaces and bracelets.

★   If you have drawer space, you can buy drawer dividers made especially for your jewellery. There are plenty to choose from that cater to all styles and budgets.

★   You can purchase decorative storage options, such as jewellery stands, if you prefer to have your jewellery on display.

By dividing your drawer(s) into sections with the dividers, you create more space than you would have without them. You can designate a section to each category of accessories.

'THE STORAGE SOLUTIONS AND SPACE-SAVING HACKS THEY HAVE INTRODUCED ME TO ARE LIFE-CHANGING! THANK YOU, GIRLS, YOU ARE THE BEST!'

Amanda Holden

CHEST OF DRAWERS

Never underestimate the power of drawer space! Drawer space is normally the home for things like your underwear, socks and tights. You can make the most of this space and keep it organised by using drawer dividers. These will separate items in clear categories, which when getting ready can be a game-changer! No more hunting for a thong amongst a sea of socks and tights!

You can store bras colour-coordinated one after the other in a row (think Victoria's Secret vibes) or if space is an issue you can fold the cups of the bra into each other and still store them in the same way, they just won't be taking up as much space. This method allows you to see everything you have and actually takes up less space than if they were left to run wild in the drawer. Use drawer dividers to then separate your tights from your socks, and your knickers from your thongs.

top tip

Make sure your drawer space is deep, with drawers that pull all the way out. This allows you to see everything that's inside and prevents anything being forgotten about at the back!

One of our upcycling transformations

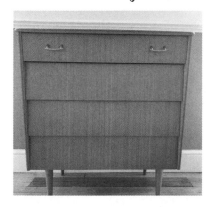 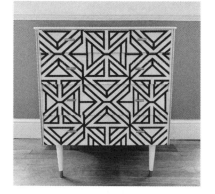

It's amazing what you can do with a lick of paint and some fresh handles! Turn to page 210 for upcycling advice to transform a piece or your overall space!

A Step by Step Guide

THE FOLD & ROLL

Drawers house all sorts of everyday clothing items and can quickly become clutter spots. This is where we like to use our fold and roll technique. This technique allows you to not only gain more space and see everything you have, but also to store sets together. You can fold and roll matching sets into each other and then place into a drawer or divide the drawer into categories and roll the items separately. The aesthetic results are stunning and folding is a very mindful, doable task, i.e. a small win when life is getting on top of you and you're keen to gain back control.

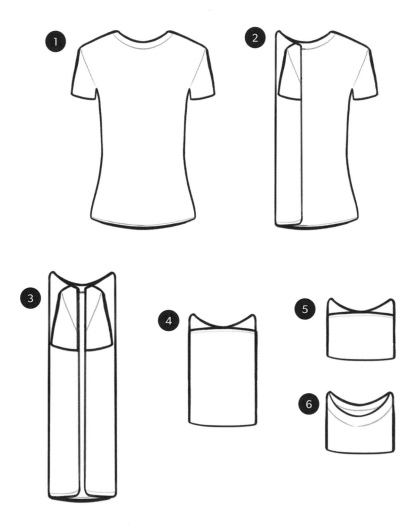

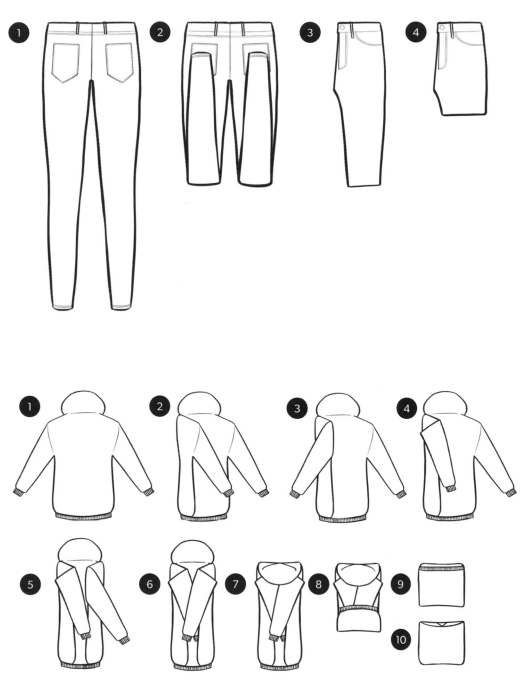

UPDATING YOUR CLOSET

Depending on your space, there are a few things you can do to refresh your wardrobe. Whether you have a smaller wardrobe or are lucky enough to have a lovely, large walk-in version (see opposite), there are ways you can personalise it that not only make it more functional but can add some style too.

Here are our tips to consider when it comes to the home of your clothes:

★ If you have doors on your wardrobe, consider updating the handles. It is amazing what a simple tweak can do to the space.

★ Selecting matching storage baskets can make everything look lovely as well as provide you with more storage – win–win!

★ Switch up the layout of your wardrobe if it's not working for you. Don't be afraid to tailor the layout to suit you. Need more hanging space? Consider adding another rail into your wardrobe. Likewise, if it's shelf space you're after, take a rail out and add in some extra shelves.

★ There are various wardrobe accessories available from most retailers that can help you make the most of your space. Hanging shelves, shoe racks and hangers that hold more than one garment are good choices, to name just a few!

★ Change your hangers! Whenever we detox and organise a wardrobe, we always recommend space-saving, slimline velvet hangers (see page 216 for where to get them). They allow you to get three hangers to every one wooden one. That's a lot of extra space! Having matching space-saving hangers will also keep your clothes looking beautiful, organised and stylish.

★ If you have the space for it, we always love to do something a little decorative in a wardrobe when we can. For example, if you have some space spare, why not make a stylish small display of things that make you happy? It could be your wedding shoes and a photo of your special day in a frame, for example. They are probably shoes you don't wear often (if at all), so having them on display is a lovely reminder of your big day.

WALK-IN WARDROBE

Designing a walk-in wardrobe for a client is one of our favourite things to do, but it can also be very challenging. If you're planning to have a walk-in wardrobe built, we have some handy tips to consider. We've lost count of the number of times we've been in a client's walk-in wardrobe and grown frustrated for them as the layout could have been designed so much better. Sometimes you can have a beautiful idea for a space, but you have to be practical and realistic about what will actually work. Every detail needs to be carefully considered.

Client Stories

We had one very high-profile client who had a wardrobe designed by a top interior designer and, while the room looked stunning, the rails for the clothes were square! The client had not yet moved into their home and when we were unpacking everything the clothes just kept falling off the rails because the square was too big, and the hangers didn't fit on. It was one of the most frustrating things we have ever experienced! Not to mention it was the hottest day of the year!

The problem people face when having a walk-in wardrobe made is that the carpenter doesn't always take into consideration their clothes and what needs to be homed in there. Whenever we are planning one for a client, the first thing we do is take thorough and in-depth notes of what needs to be stored there. Do they have lots of shoes and bags or are there more clothes? Would they benefit from more shelves, rails or drawers? What are their buying habits when it comes to their wardrobe? How do they like their items arranged? What layout works best for their lifestyle? These are all things you should be asking yourself when planning this space. The single most important thing is making sure this space is going to be perfect for YOU. Yes, you want it to look beautiful, but ultimately you won't care how lovely it is if it doesn't fit everything in and isn't flowing in a calm, practical and seamless way, especially as walk-in wardrobes can be an expensive undertaking.

TOP TIPS
for a stylish walk-in wardrobe

★ Look at the space and make sure you're making the most of it with the layout. Do you need more rail space or shelf space? Try to maximise both, if you can.

★ Think about rail height! You don't want your clothes hitting the rail below and equally you don't want your clothes on the lower rail pooling on the base of the wardrobe/floor.

★ Most people want a full-length mirror in their dressing area. Ideally you don't want to lose any wall space to a mirror, so either consider mirrored doors or look at placing a mirror on the inside of the door as you walk in. If you're having an open wardrobe with no doors but shelving space, consider a secret cupboard which looks as though it's a mirror, but you can open it and there is shelving behind. You could even have one large sliding mirror.

★ If you want an island in the middle of the room, drawers always work well in these. Some people like to have the top open, and then you can have your accessories on display. This can look lovely but take into consideration how much jewellery you have and whether or not you will keep it tidy – you could end up with a messy drawer on display!

★ Storage ottomans are a great feature to add to a wardrobe and they can really finish the space off nicely. They look lovely, give you somewhere to sit and you can store things in them.

★ Accent chairs can help to give a walk-in wardrobe a boutique feel. These work for any size of dressing room.

★ Consider taking any radiators off. This isn't a big job and will again help you maximise space.

★ If you are planning on turning a former room into a wardrobe, sometimes you may come up against the obstacles of windows or a radiator which could throw you when planning the space. A top tip when planning this room is blocking the window. While it is lovely having some natural light, it isn't the end of the world to lose it in a walk-in wardrobe. A simple hack is to put a blind up in the window and leave it permanently down, then place the frame of the wardrobe in front. It looks absolutely fine from outside and on the inside, you would never know there was a window there. This is an inexpensive way of maximising space!

★ If you are planning on placing a dressing table in this room, place this under the window so you don't lose any wardrobe space. Placing a mirror in front of the window won't block any light coming into the room and will also be the perfect spot for you to do your make-up.

★ If you have wall space or a shelf, add artwork/photo frames to personalise the space and make you smile.

★ Long, vertical shelving is an interesting way to display decorative items in a walk-in wardrobe. You could pair artwork with a special pair of shoes and a lovely diffuser for example. It can be something small that gives a little bit of wow factor.

★ We always recommend adding LED strips to a walk-in wardrobe. Not only are you able to see everything a little better but it makes it feel that bit more luxe.

DOORS OR NO DOORS?

We are often asked whether it is better to have doors on a wardrobe or not as people can sometimes be concerned about things getting dusty in an open wardrobe. There's no right or wrong answer here; it can depend on the space and what you feel will work best for you. We both love the look of each version and both come with their own small list of pros and cons.

Below are some points to consider for each:

With doors

★ *It won't matter as much if your wardrobe gets a little messy.*

★ *Provides the perfect opportunity to add mirrors to the space.*

★ *Can look tidier.*

★ *Adding doors to a walk-in wardrobe will bump up the cost.*

★ *You don't see everything you have at once.*

★ *Your items won't gather as much dust.*

★ *Sliding doors can be awkward as there is always one section you can't see.*

★ *If it's a narrow room they can take up too much space.*

Without doors

★ *You can see everything more clearly.*

★ *Your walk-in won't be as expensive to build.*

★ *You can feel more inspired when it comes to putting outfits together.*

★ *Items, especially shoes, can sometimes get a little dusty in an open wardrobe but this is nothing a feather duster can't fix!*

★ *If it gets messy, it's all on show!*

★ *Doesn't take up as much space.*

Use two hangers to help make one long item shorter in length. Place a long maxi dress, for example, on a hanger, then place the end of the dress through the second hanger and then hang them up together. This will prevent longer items getting in the way, and is especially helpful if you don't have any or many long hanging rails.

top tip

For smaller walk-in wardrobes we recommend no doors as they can take up too much space, be awkward and make smaller rooms feel even smaller. Just make sure you keep on top of the organising to ensure it is looking its very best.

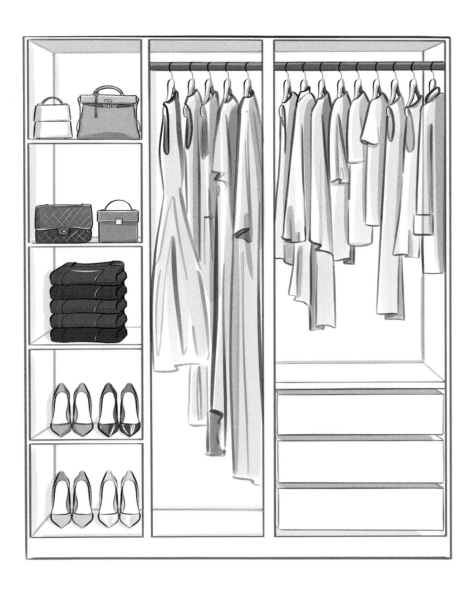

CREATING A STAPLE WARDROBE

We cannot recommend building a good staple wardrobe enough. The perfect capsule wardrobe is a collection of good-quality and timeless pieces. These clothes and shoes are not fast fashion, and they are not 'in fashion'. They do not go in and out of style – they are classic items that are the foundation of the way you get dressed and style things up.

Having a fail-safe staple wardrobe will not only help you always have something to wear, but you can then be really selective about what items you let into your wardrobe after this! This is especially beneficial if you're struggling with your sense of style and finding it hard to choose outfits to wear despite seeming to have a wardrobe overflowing with clothes.

Try to be strict about what you let into your wardrobe. Don't just buy something because it is in the sale (this can often to lead to purchase regret throughout the home, not just in the wardrobe – we've all been there!) or because it's cheap, especially if you only 'kind of' like it. No matter how expensive or cheap an item is, only allow it to come home with you if you love it and will wear it. Think of your wardrobe like a party – you only want people you love there!

Always, always try stuff on. Be realistic about when and how you're going to wear it and pay attention to how it makes you feel. Doing this before allowing any item into your wardrobe prevents buyer's remorse.

The perfect capsule wardrobe is a collection of good-quality and timeless pieces. These clothes and shoes are not fast fashion, and they are not 'in fashion'.

STYLE SISTERS
must-haves

The following pieces are an investment and should be well thought out. Take the time to get these items right and we promise you will have the perfect foundation for creating a stylish and functional wardrobe.

These are pieces that can be dressed up or down and that will remain so for years to come!

DENIM JEANS

Denim was first introduced in 1873 and we honestly wonder what people did before this – can you imagine your wardrobe with no denim? Having a pair of well-fitted, comfortable jeans in your wardrobe will be one of your best investments. Jeans have the power to make an outfit and can be worn dressed up or down.

BLAZER

This piece should be well fitted and not mimic something you would buy for the office! You can wear a blazer dressed up or it can be worn more casually. It's a versatile piece that, once invested in, would be deeply missed when gone! Pair with a T-shirt, jeans and trainers for a laid-back and stylish look or with a smarter top and high heels for the evening.

WHITE T-SHIRT

Staple white t-shirts are the perfect classic piece that can be subtly accessorised with scarves and simple or statement jewellery.

LEATHER JACKET

A great-fitting, classic PU/leather jacket is something that rarely, if ever, goes out of style. Sticking to a classic shape means it will remain in your wardrobe forever.

DENIM JACKET

Perfect to layer under coats or with chunky knitwear in the winter, or to wear on its own in the warmer months. The same rules apply as for a leather jacket. Go for a classic, well-fitting style and this will stay with you for many years to come!

SHIRT

A classic white shirt that can be worn alone or under a jumper is an item you will likely turn to on many occasions. You can dress it up or down. Look for a version with a trendy vibe, it might have a decorative button or be slightly oversized. The fabric should feel a lot nicer than a typical office/school shirt.

Don't ever underestimate the power of a perfect white T!

BLOUSE
No wardrobe is complete without a pretty blouse! This can be in black, white or any bold print. As long as you keep the shape quite classic, it will stay in your staple wardrobe forever.

CAMI
Remember that blazer we mentioned? Pairing a cami with a blazer, jeans/trousers and heels will instantly give you a classic and stylish outfit for that last-minute night out – we've all been there! This look doesn't date so it's a must when it comes to your staple wardrobe.

VEST
Great-quality, fitted vests are a lifeline in your wardrobe. You can wear them alone, layered, dressed up or down. When you find the perfect one, we recommend buying it in all the colours and even doubling up on the black and white staples.

MATCHING LOUNGE SUIT
We.all.need.one. You will always need one. Is your wardrobe even a wardrobe if you don't have one?! There are plenty of styles available for you to find the perfect version for you. You want it to be comfy enough to throw on at home but nice enough to run to the shops in.

DAY-TO-NIGHT MIDI DRESS
This is an item you want to buy in the shape that suits your figure best. Keep it plain so that it doesn't date. This way you can keep it on trend over the years and change it up with different accessories.

BLACK BOOTS
Black biker boots, knee-highs and plain ankle boots will always pair well with any outfit.

SMART TRAINERS
Pair with a blazer and jeans, or even a casual dress.

BAGS
A classic-shaped tote and clutch will always perfectly accessorise any look. Consider buying in classic black, nude or even red. These colours will go with any outfit.

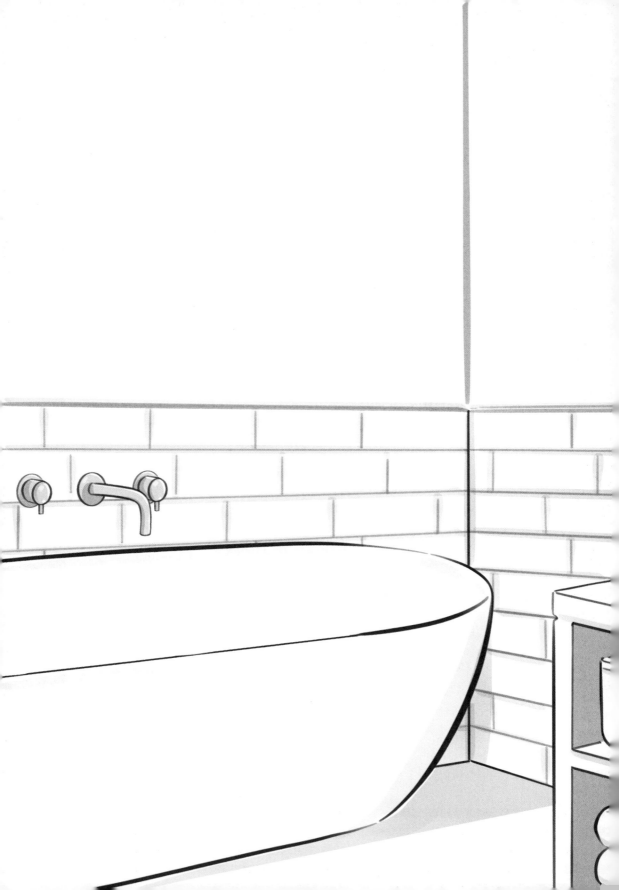

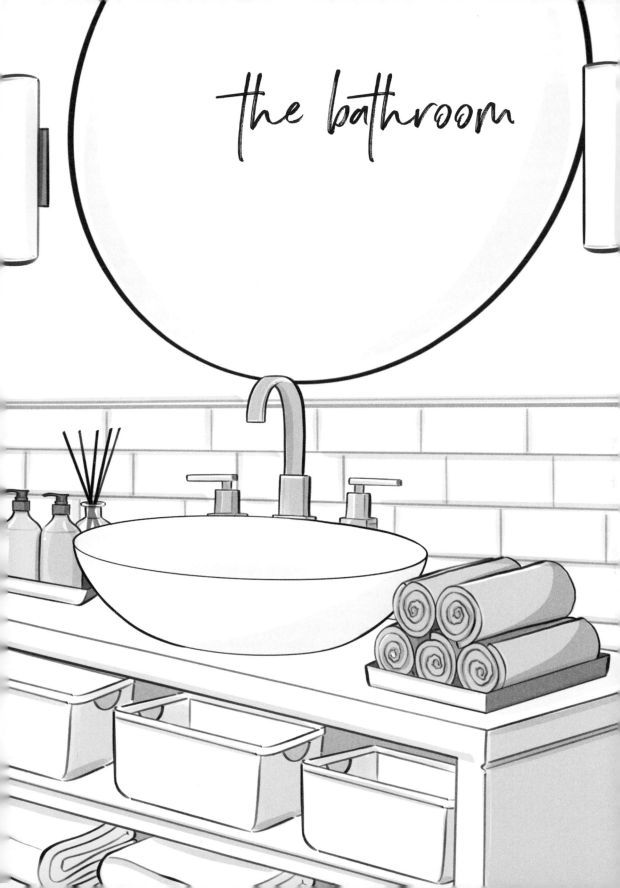

the bathroom

the bathroom

SOAK, RELAX & UNWIND

The bathroom often gets overlooked when it comes to its practicality and usage. It is a hub of activity and can become full of mess in a matter of minutes, so it's crucial to try and add some harmony and optimise space and organisation.

Your bathroom should feel clean, fresh and clutter-free so you can move around easily without tripping over things or feeling overwhelmed by colourful products all over the place. There is no better feeling than running a nice warm bath, lighting a few candles and unwinding with a lovely soak, especially in the cold winter months.

Firstly, you need to detox your bathroom following the steps we laid out for you in The Process on pages 36–9. As with other rooms in the house, you don't want anything here that doesn't belong or would make more sense homed elsewhere. The bathroom should only be home to items such as:

★ **washing products**: shower gel, bubble bath and shampoo/ conditioner
★ **hand wash and hand cream**
★ **body products**: creams, lotions and gels
★ **medicine** (make sure it's high up and out of reach if there are children in the house)
★ **bath toys**, if you have children (remember to clean toys regularly as they can go mouldy inside)
★ **towels**
★ **candles/diffuser**
★ **spare toilet rolls**
★ **bathroom cleaning products** (if you have the space to store)
★ **excess/extra products** (if you have the space to store)

The way to work out your categories is to get everything out. Make piles of products and what they are used for, check their dates and how much is left in them. Can they be decanted into a larger container? Do you have excess amounts of the same item? And the most important question – do you use the item/product? If the answer is no, don't put it back. Give it away to a friend or family member or bin it and recycle the packaging if you can. You can then group similar products together for storing. For instance, you could have a hair container for shampoo, conditioners and hair masks, and a face container for face washes, face masks and treatments.

Consider what items can be removed from their original packaging and transferred into glass jars or acrylic or ceramic containers. This will give your bathroom a more streamlined and stylish look. You can also make your own labels using your label machine (see page 31)!

WHAT GOES WHERE?

Showers should be a clear space with only the products you are using in there. No empty shampoo bottles taking up valuable floor space; only use the shower to home products that you are going to use.

If you have a vanity unit around the sink area, this is ideal for an under-the-sink storage unit or it may already have shelves inside it. In this case it's all about adding storage containers and sectioning items in their relevant categories. If you have drawers under your sink or a cupboard, the same rules apply – use drawer dividers to split the space into categories and this way everything will stay in its relevant place. This stops you from buying excess products and helps you to use up everything you have before buying more. Don't forget to use the empty space behind the cupboard door. This is perfect for using stick-on door containers, which are great for holding products. Just remember to check the door still closes once it's stuck on!

If you have an open shelving unit or a freestanding one without doors, you can get nice decorative storage containers to put away your products in or display neatly on the shelf in category order. Adding open shelving to the wall is a good option, no matter the layout or size of your space. Everyone will have empty walls in their bathroom that can be utilised. Using the space above the toilet is also a popular choice, or above the doorway if you have space. You can make these display shelves to put decorative products and items on to add to interest to the room or add woven baskets as a neat storage solution. If open shelving isn't your thing, a wall-mounted cabinet is another option for extra storage. Using stick-on 3M Command™ hooks is a simple way to hang up hairdryers, straighteners and curlers behind a cupboard door. This way they will stay neat and tangle-free if you wrap the wire around the appliance before you hang it up.

TOP TIPS for a stylish bathroom

★ **CALMING COLOURS**
We love bathrooms to be fresh, clean and simple with clean lines and plenty of light. But the bathroom is also a room where you can inject some colour and add personality, for example having dusky pink tiles around the sink area and then using the same colour but in a different shaped tile inside the shower area. This keeps the bathroom in sync but using different shapes and styles of tiles adds that extra interest.

★ **RE-GROUT & REFRESH**
If your bathroom is looking a little tired and needs a bit of an update but you are on a budget, consider re-grouting the tiles. This can make a big difference to the overall look of the room and you can even get grout pens that you can use to colour in the grout to make it look fresh and new. If you fancy going one step further, try painting your bathroom tiles. There are lots of tile paints out there, and you may need to put a primer on before you paint, so check the paint instructions before you start. This will definitely give the bathroom a new lease of life! These small adjustments can make such a difference to your home.

★ **UPDATE YOUR FLOOR**
If the floor tiles or lino are looking a bit worn out, replacing it will instantly make the bathroom look newer. A little freshen up of any paint work will work wonders too!

★ **THINK ABOUT LIGHTING**
Lighting in a bathroom is important – make sure any option you choose is suitable for the steamy conditions. Remember bright light and clean lines are a must-have! Wall lights work well in a bathroom or a backlit mirror is also a great addition which adds ambience.

★ **MIRROR, MIRROR**
A backlit wall mirror or freestanding mirror with a light is handy for doing your make-up or any close-up face work, such as plucking your eyebrows.

★ **TOP TOWELS**
You can create a spa-like vibe in your bathroom by making towels a feature. Roll and place them on shelves and make sure they are all matching colours and/or styles otherwise they can look messy.

Small hand towels placed beside the sink with a little basket to throw the dirty ones in can also introduce a hotel/spa feel in your own home. It does add to the washing load, so you can always replace them with paper hand towels and a bin to throw the used tissue away in if you'd prefer.

★ **STYLISH ACCESSORIES**
Bathroom accessories are key to styling the space – a nice bath mat and matching towels around the room will give it a simple yet stylish look. We love white towels as they're so fresh and clean looking, but if your bathroom is a neutral palette and you fancy adding a pop of colour to the room with the towels you can be more experimental.

★ **DISPENSER DELIGHT**
Hand soap and hand lotion placed into matching dispensers adds a luxury vibe to your bathroom. Remember to keep the accent metal tones the same, so if your taps are chrome be sure to get a chrome pump dispenser, so it all matches and looks like a family of products.

★ **ADD SOME GREENERY**
Houseplants love a bathroom, and they soak up the humidity and moisture in the room after a steamy shower or bath – aloe vera and bird's nest fern are great options. Placed in a nice pot or stand, plants will add colour and life to the room. (See page 206 for our favourite houseplants.)

★ **FRESH FRAGRANCE**
Fragrance is so important in a bathroom – you want an uplifting scent that will disguise any bathroom odours and make you feel energised and awake when getting prepped for the day. Get a matching room spray to spritz the room when needed!

the small bathroom

If you are short on space in your bathroom, the simplest way to gain extra storage is to use the walls. Get wall-mounted shelves or cupboards – this is essential for storing all your products, medicines and bathroom cleaning products. Choose a wall-mounted cabinet with mirrored doors as this provides practical storage as well as a handy mirror.

A bath shelf is another multipurpose item as it can sit over the bath to store your products or provide a surface for a drink or book when you're relaxing in the tub, and when not in use it can home a stylish candle. If you have a bit of floor space, a ladder shelf is a great option.

If you like to keep your products in the shower, consider purchasing a shower caddy to store all of your items for easy access when showering.

Towel rails are lovely to hang towels and even better if they are heated to warm them up to use after showering or bathing. Make sure that the towel rail matches the décor of the room as you don't want it looking out of place or ruin the clean aesthetic.

If you have a separate toilet and sink in a small room like a cloakroom, consider using a wallpaper in here. We love it when people use a bold print in a small room. Don't be afraid to get adventurous with your design – it's a great little room to inject with a bit of personality!

the large bathroom

The beauty of a larger bathroom is the luxury of space and being able to home more items in the room. If you have the space on top of your vanity sink unit, bathroom trays are a nice way to add a decorative touch to the space. Place a candle or diffuser, mini plant, or your soap dispenser on the tray (see more on page 171).

If you have a freestanding bath, consider having a little bench, stool or chair near it as a decorative but practical item of furniture. You can place clothing on there for before or after your bath/shower or place a drink or candle on there if it's a flat stool.

If you have the space in a cupboard or under the sink, it's handy to have a caddy of bathroom cleaning essentials, such as cloths and sprays for easy access. If all items are placed together in a caddy with a handle it's simple to pick them up and put back when needed.

top tip

When choosing your bathroom storage containers, make sure they are water-resistant or waterproof so they keep in the best possible condition and/or can be easily wiped cleaned if you spill some liquid on them.

Handy reminder: The Process

TO-DO CHECKLIST

The following can be applied whether you are tackling an area at a time or completing the whole room at once:

- ☐ **Get everything out** of the cupboards/drawers
- ☐ **Check the dates**
- ☐ **Detox and organise into three piles:** keep, chuck, donate/give to friends or family
- ☐ **Purchase** new storage containers
- ☐ **Put the keep items into categories**, i.e. body creams, medicines, shampoos
- ☐ **Label** the containers or storage boxes
- ☐ **Decant** smaller products into larger containers. If you have two of the same shampoos and one has a bit left in it, pour that into one of the containers. Be resourceful and use up products before opening new ones

WHAT YOU NEED CHECKLIST

- ☐ bin bags
- ☐ vacuum cleaner
- ☐ cleaning products
- ☐ storage containers/boxes
- ☐ label machine/labels

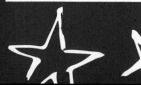

The Style Sisters
guide to styling your . . .

bathroom tray

Bring hotel glam vibes to your bathroom by adding a tray to your sink, vanity area or a shelf. Having a neat and stylish tray will add that little extra sparkle to your bathroom. Collate items in a similar colour palette that works well with your bathroom tones and style. Pieces on your tray can be decorative and/or practical, such as:

1. HAND SOAP/LOTION
Decant into matching dispensers for that luxe feel.

2. DIFFUSERS AND/OR CANDLE
Choose an uplifting fragrance that will energise or relax you, depending on what vibe you're after.

3. SMALL SUCCULENT PLANT
To add a pop of colour and life to the room.

4. TRINKET TRAY
To keep jewellery in when bathing or showering.

Turn to page 162 to see our sample illustration in action.

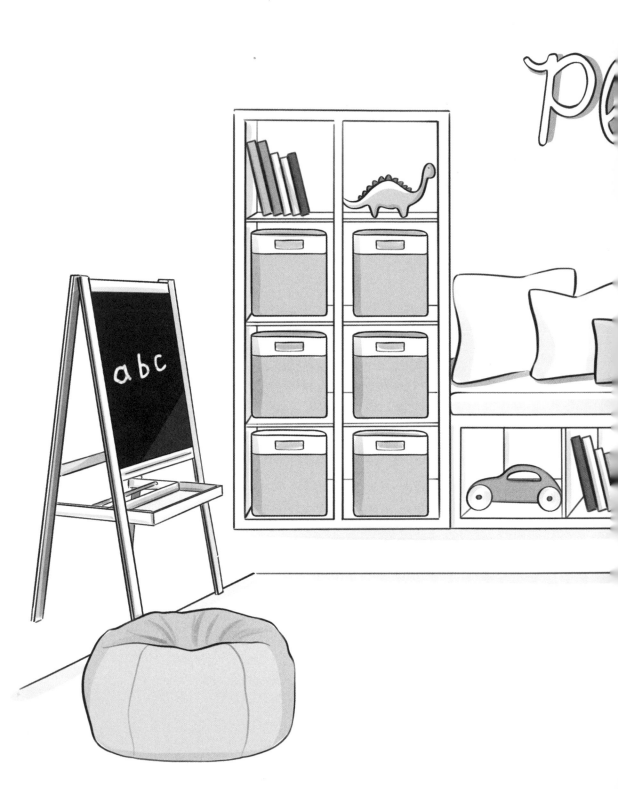

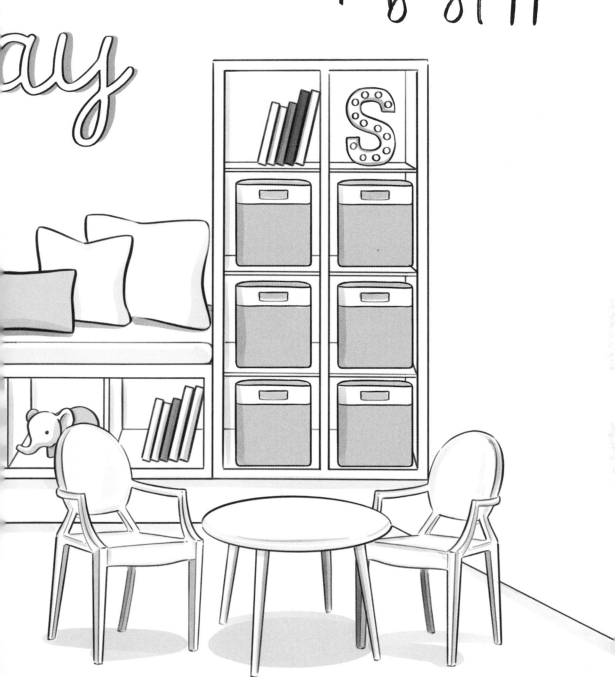

kids' stuff

kids' stuff

TOYS, TOYS EVERYWHERE...
LET'S FIND THEM A HOME!

If you're reading this chapter, it means you have children, and we all know what comes with kids – toys, and lots of them! It's OK, don't panic, we will help you find super savvy and stylish ways of storing these brightly coloured pieces.

So where do the toys currently live? A playroom? Your child's bedroom? The living room? Or basically all over the house?! It's time to bring some order and organisation to the toy situation. You don't want to become the evil parent who has hidden all the fun toys away so that the house looks nice and tidy, but you do want practical storage and places for the toys to live when they are not being played with. If you don't have a designated room for your children to play in and home all the toys, there are some really clever and practical ways in which they can be stored away so when you are chilling on the sofa you won't spot a Peppa Pig staring up at you from the floor. It's your home and it can be an equally adult- and child-friendly space – you don't have to feel guilty about wanting to hide toys away when the kids are in bed and it's time for the house to regain full adult mode for a few short hours!

WHILE THE KIDS ARE AWAY...
The first thing you are going to do is have a toy detox! It's important to do this when your children are at nursery, school or just not around. We can assure you that they will want to keep everything, and the detox process will not go very well!

Follow the steps we laid out for you in The Process on pages 36–9. Be realistic about what toys your child currently plays with. We all know that they outgrow and go off characters quickly and they all love a fad. We have been there – your child is into a certain character one month, so you buy lots of toys and then all of a sudden, they are on to the next best thing. Donate or give toys away as long as they are in good working order; it's a wonderful feeling to give toys to children who you know are going to play with and get lots of enjoyment from them.

Children like to collect tat – it's a fact! Party-bag plastic toys, characters that comes with meals or in food packets, and random items from day trips can all make their way into the ever-expanding toy collection, so it's time to get things straight and get rid of items that have accumulated in the toy section just because they had nowhere else to go. It's OK to chuck items out, recycle where you can and donate. (Remember to take out any batteries and recycle them at your local supermarket.)

If children seem to only play with certain toys, we often recommend to our clients to rotate their toy collection. Split their toys into two groups and store one group away, then bring them back out after a few months and swap them with the toys they are playing with. This way your children will feel like they are getting new toys and they are more likely to want to play with them, rather than them just sitting forgotten about in a cupboard.

STORAGE SOLUTIONS

Storage baskets are a practical way to store toys. You can get them in a variety of styles, fabrics, textures and colours. Make sure they are child-friendly and that your child can easily get toys in and out of them – you can train them to be tidy and organised from a young age! Storage boxes or baskets with handles are a good idea as they are easier to take on and off shelves or storage units – be careful that nothing too heavy is up high to avoid accidents.

IKEA is an excellent, affordable place to shop for storage solutions for children's playrooms or storage for toys around the house. The KALLAX system is one of our favourites. You can design different layouts with it to suit your space – we love to build a storage seating area by creating a U shape out of the units and making the middle section a seating area by adding cushions. We have used this design in lots of our clients' houses and it looks great and is really practical. You can even get creative and spray the units different colours and then customise the storage baskets that go inside – this is a fab way to design something unique.

We love to use clear acrylic storage boxes by iDesign in a kid's room; not only are they stackable, which is amazing when you have a tall cupboard shelf, but they help you to maximise space as you can stack another storage box on top of the initial one – so two boxes full of toys instead of one. Acrylic storage is also a clever way to store smaller toy figures and arts and crafts supplies, and children can easily see what's inside the box, so its contents don't get forgotten about and so less junk accumulates...

We always label the boxes so that the toys can go back where they belong, and it instills a sense of order to the room. One fun way of doing this is adding a picture of the item that's inside – you could print off a sticker of a car and your child will then know that the toy cars go in that box. It can be a fun game and you could make it a race against time or give them a little treat once they have tidied everything up at the end of the day.

Client Stories

A popular hack that we used for our client Stacey Solomon was dividing her son's LEGO into acrylic storage boxes by colour. This took us five hours to complete, including battling a box of LEGO men falling down the stairs and a bad back, but the results were AMAZING! It looked so visually pleasing with all the beautiful bright colours all in their correct compartments, all lined up in the cupboard. We were thrilled. This organising hack inspired many mums and dads out there to do the same with their children's LEGO and toy bricks. It also helps children to find exactly what type of LEGO they need as it's all colour-coordinated!

If storing board games, jigsaw puzzles and other games that come in large boxes is taking up too much space and you've got limited places to home them, remove them from the boxes and place them in zip-up wallets. You can get these in different sizes and colours. Put the pieces, instructions and box front, if it's a puzzle, inside the wallet and label the front so that you know what is inside. You can then store these efficiently by popping them in a storage box or on a shelf: reduced packaging = more space!

We also love using an acrylic lazy Susan as it has compartments which can house pens, pencils and arts and crafts bits in an organised way. It can also look really fun and can be left on a table as a feature, and it's super practical as it spins around and is easy for children to grab what they want.

A storage cart on wheels is a great way to store creative items like paints, pens, paper, colouring books, etc. These can all be contained in the cart and wheeled around to where they are needed. We found one of the best ones available is from IKEA, and it can also be sprayed in a colour to suit the look of the room. Storage boxes on wheels are another practical way of storing toys as these can also be wheeled around to wherever the children are playing and then put back out of the way at the end of the day.

Hanging pots don't have to be used only for plants and herbs in the kitchen; they are also a fun way to store pens, pencils, crayons and brushes. Place on hooks along a rail so they can hang at a child-friendly height. If you have a creative/art table, then try to place them alongside this so they are near where they will be used.

Sometimes there are some toys that just can't be stored away and hidden, unless you have a giant storage cupboard. Yes, we are talking about the Barbie DreamHouse, a doll's house or castle. In this case you have to just make these display pieces and decorate the room with them – use these toys to line the edges of the room. This is a space for your children to play and be imaginative – if every toy is hidden it wouldn't be a place to play!

If your little one likes to collect soft toys and has a teddy collection that looks like a toy shop, it can be a nightmare to find somewhere to store them! There are a few practical ways these can be stored out of the way. One clever hack is to get a giant bean bag, take out the beans inside and instead stuff the bag with the soft toys. This way your child can sit on the bean (teddy) bag and then when they want to play with them just unzip, empty and play! Alternatively you can add a teddy zoo, a freestanding decorative piece of furniture that houses all your children's soft toys. They can see through the bars and easily pull the teddy they want out of there. This is perfect if your child has lots of teddies!

Over-the-door fabric shoe storage can also be used to store soft toys, action figures and dolls. Behind doors is a great unused space that should always be utilised if you're short on space.

If your kids love to dress up and you have lots of fancy dress stuff, a kid-friendly clothes rail is ideal teamed with kids' velvet hangers to hang items on. Don't forget you can get more on the rail with slimline hangers (see page 152)! You could create a little fancy-dress area, clothes rail and storage basket filled with dressing up pieces to make a kids' dressing up heaven!

TOP TIPS for a playful space

★ **PRINTS & POSTERS**

Kids' rooms should definitely have an element of fun in them. A simple way of doing this is by adding artwork in frames. These can be easily changed as your kids grow older and they are a cheaper way of decorating a room than wallpapering. This is also a great idea for a unisex room. You can use different art that appeals to all the children. Alternatively, there are stick-on wall murals that can be easily peeled off when they want a change. You can pick up some really lovely designs from Etsy and other online retailers.

Use your children's artwork as a feature in a playroom. If they have some amazing masterpieces, why not get them framed or put up a big moodboard of images on a wall of all their creativity? This can be easily updated with new pieces of art just by pinning up new creations or replacing older pieces with more recent efforts.

top tip

If your little ones are very creative and love to draw and paint and you don't have the heart to chuck their creations away, you can quickly build up an out-of-control pile of paper full of scribbles and paint! Our ingenious solution for this is to take a picture of each artwork and collate all the photos for a year in one place. You can then get a photo book printed online of your children's masterpieces and title the book 'Artwork 2021' or similar. This way members of the family and your child can enjoy looking back over the pics in an easy-to-store photo book.

This is a lovely thing to then store in their memory box or you can pick out favourite drawings and store the originals in there if you want to keep one or two.

★ **PRACTICAL FLOORING**

Flooring is important in a playroom – it needs to be practical, wipeable, easy to clean and not too fluffy or shaggy! Carpet can be nice and soft for children to play on but do make sure the pile is short as you don't want tiny bits of LEGO getting stuck in the carpet.

The same rule applies to rugs – short flat pile is the best type to put in a high-traffic playing zone. Invest in a wipe clean playmat for when your child is using things like paints or Play-Doh so that you can protect the floor!

★ **ADVENTUROUS DESIGN**

You can be a little more adventurous with the design in a playroom or a child's bedroom. You can make it fun and playful by adding textures and accessorising with fun cushions, wall prints and lettering around the room. Make it personal by adding the child's name or use their initials to make the room unique to them and so it feels like it's their space.

★ **TOP TABLE**

If you have the space for a child-friendly table and chairs, these are a must. Not only can your little one sit at their own small table but they can play, draw and be creative on it. It also looks really cute in a playroom.

A desk/study zone is also lovely in a playroom area. You can keep educational books, computers or laptops nearby and this can be used as the key focused area where your child does school work at home.

★ **READING NOOK**

Try creating a little reading nook in the corner of the room. A small tepee tent or canopy can be hung or put up to make a little area especially for reading. Adding fairy lights can make it feel dreamy and calm. Place some bookshelves, a bookcase or storage basket of books nearby so they are accessible. Don't forget to add cushions and blankets to make it super comfy.

Not only can this reading nook look super cute, but it's a functional area that can be used by the whole family to chill and read together.

★ **BRILLIANT BLACKBOARD**
A blackboard is always a nice feature in a toy room and encourages your little ones to get creative in their own space. It's practical as it can be easily wiped clean and you can even get magnetic blackboard paint, so magnets can also be placed on the wall – this is hours of fun for your little ones! We designed this look for Rochelle and Marvin Humes in the toy room of their new home and this should be a modern, fun and imaginative space for the kids to enjoy for many years to come.

★ **LIGHT IT UP**
If you like the look of neon lights, this is a vibrant touch to add to a toy room. You can get any quote, name or saying that you can think of made for a really personal look. Choose your font, colour and style of neon for a cool update for your toy room!

Rochelle Humes' playroom

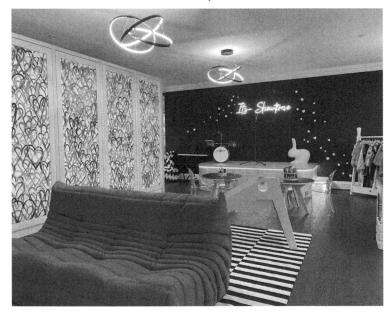

Client Stories

We absolutely loved creating Rochelle and Marvin Humes' playroom and it's one of our favourite rooms we have designed to date. We worked closely with our very talented carpenter to build some beautiful, bespoke, deep wall cupboard units that had a stunning curve to them. They were so deep we could both stand in them with room to move and these were specially designed by us to hide and home all of the larger doll's houses and prams.

When adding storage in your home it's crucial to work out what you want to use it for and if those items will actually fit, right from the get-go. We knew that we wanted Rochelle and Marvin to be able to store these large toys away, so we had to create storage that was big enough for them. We designed the front of these units with custom spray-painted art panels that can be changed in the future if the theme of the room changes. They added something really fun and interesting to the space and made the most feature. Being able to change the panels was important to us; children grow and so do their interests, so when decorating or styling a playroom (or child's bedroom) think about how the room can grow with your child. If they are into a certain character at the moment, they may be into something else by the time the room is finished, so keep it fairly neutral and add in characters and colours with the accessories.

Our favourite part was the curved performance stage which had steps leading up to it with clever storage drawers underneath and lighting. With any space you have think about how it can be used for storage – there was no point having a hollow stage with wasted space underneath, so it made perfect sense to add drawers. We placed musical instruments on the stage including drums as well as a microphone and it really came alive with the addition of a magnetic blackboard wall behind the stage with a cool neon light glowing the words 'It's showtime'. The room just screamed fun, playful and stylish, we both definitely released our inner child!

'MY STYLE SISTERS GEMMA AND CHARLOTTE, I'D BE KNEE-DEEP IN EXCESS IF IT WEREN'T FOR YOU TWO CLEVER LADIES! YOU HELPED ME UNCLUTTER MY PANTRY WHICH LED ME TO UNCLUTTER MY LIFE! CAN'T WAIT TO USE YOU AGAIN, YOU ARE THE BEST!'

Michelle Visage

'THERE IS NO JOB TOO BIG FOR THESE GIRLS!'

Vicky Pattison

the small space

If your toy room is a part of your living room, you want to be able to zone the room (see page 63). You can do this by having furniture that has storage and cupboard space combined, for example your TV media unit might have cupboards below it or on either side to house toys and storage boxes of toys, that can be brought out when needed.

Choose a sofa footstool with a lid for another place to store toys. You really have to think about everything in the room and if there is an empty void or storage compartment then try to use it in the most practical way.

the large space

Having a larger playroom allows your imagination to run wild and provides an exciting place for children to let loose. We love to feature an area dedicated to reading and somewhere to store books as we think it's so important for little ones to enjoy the opportunity to get comfy and get lost in a book, with or without their parents involved. You can create this easily by having a bookcase or bookshelves with books on display. A canopy that hangs from the ceiling or a tepee tent filled with lots of cosy cushions is a perfect little reading hideaway (see page 179). An alternative option is a giant bean bag; you can purchase these in lots of colours, fabric and textures – just make sure it goes with the overall look of the room. Our top tip is to always order more beans to fill up the bag than you think you need as the bean bag literally eats them up so quickly!

A sofa or seating area for watching TV or gaming is also a great addition to a playroom if you have older kids and don't want PlayStations invading the adult living room. We are mums of boys, so we are familiar with all of this, and can vouch that adding a gaming zone in a playroom is priceless!

We have always loved interesting features in a playroom like a bubble chair or swing hanging from the ceiling. These are quirky, cool elements that kids go bananas for.

Handy reminder: The Process

TO-DO CHECKLIST

☐ **Detox** the toys

☐ **Create** two groups of toys that can be rotated if desired

☐ **Group** similar toys together

☐ **Contain** in storage baskets

☐ Label

WHAT YOU NEED CHECKLIST

☐ bin bags

☐ vacuum cleaner

☐ cleaning products

☐ storage containers/boxes

☐ label machine/labels

The Style Sisters
guide to styling your . . .
children's space

When styling and organising your little one's space, it is important to consider the design and style of the room, making sure that there are storage options for all their toys and making it an area that is practical and fun for your child to play in and enjoy.

1. MATCHING STORAGE BASKETS
Keeping storage baskets matching and child-friendly with soft handles is an important factor to think about when purchasing storage baskets for a toy room or kids' space.

2. DECORATIVE TOYS
We love to break up storage spaces, shelves and window ledges with decorative toys. Choose items that work well with the decor and theme of the room and add a bit of personality to the space!

3. PERSONALISED ITEMS
A nice way to personalise the space is to add initials or your child's/children's names to the room to make them feel like it's their own space. You can do this with wooden letters, artwork or neon lights.

4. CHILD SIZE FURNITURE
A desk, table and chairs or a little sofa placed in the room is a nice touch for your little ones. Remember to make sure they are washable and easily wipeable.

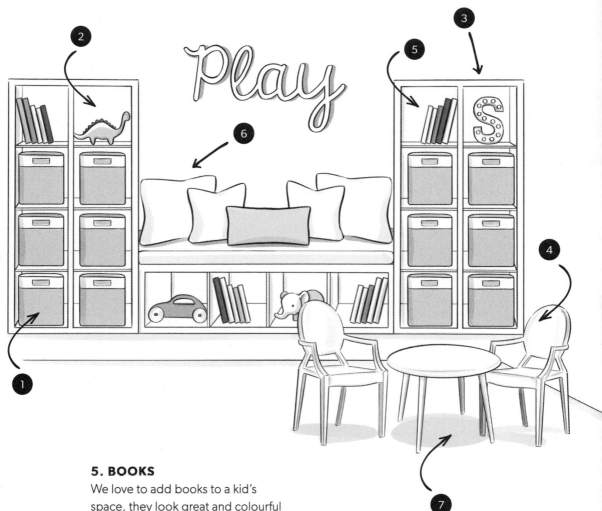

5. BOOKS

We love to add books to a kid's space, they look great and colourful on a shelf and are educational – double tick!

6. CUSHIONS/BEAN BAGS

Super fun and comfy, plus extra seating for when friends are over. Make sure they are washable in case of any spillages!

7. SHORT PILED RUGS

Rugs add texture and softness to the floor, but remember to go short-piled as anything long or fluffy will be messy in a few hours and lost toy pieces will be forgotten about forever!

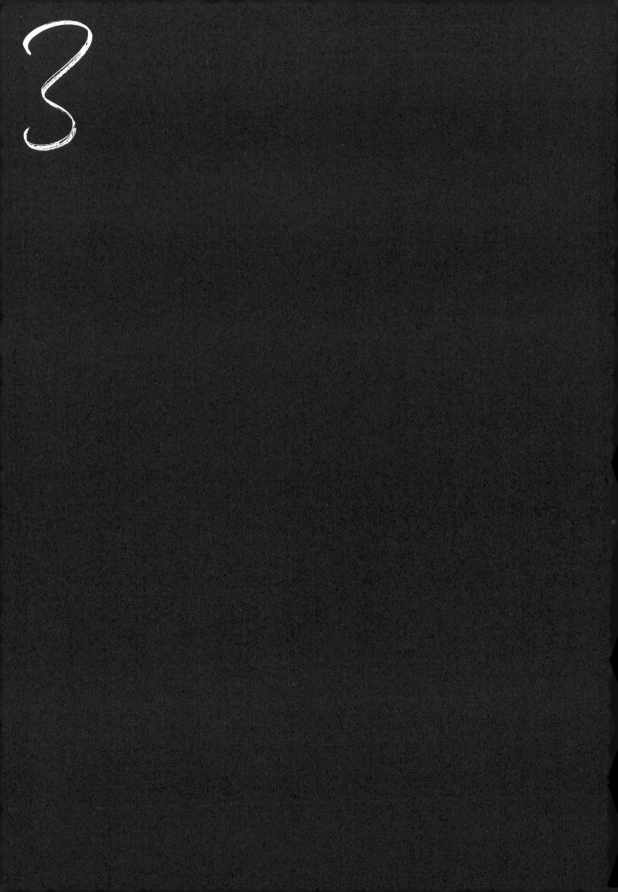

3

KEEP IT
IN CHECK

& STYLE
YOUR SPACE

STOP THE CLUTTER CREEP

We're always getting people saying 'your clients won't keep that tidy' or the classic 'that will be a mess by next week'. However, we find it happens to be the complete opposite. With our detox and organise, we give our clients a home for every single item that makes sense and works for them, so the structure stays in place for months and years after we've left. They become addicted to keeping up the effort and trusting the process. The new sense of clarity enables them to feel more in control and thrive in their homes.

It makes us so happy when we follow up with clients after a couple of months and ask how they are finding their newly organised space. We have a pretty much 100% success rate – they tell us that they are so happy that everything has a place to live. They're cleverly utilising their belongings and life seems that little bit less stressful. Being in their house has become an enjoyable experience again.

KEEP AN EYE ON IT

If after a few months you're finding things starting to get a little messy or feel like the clutter has begun to creep back in, we have some top tips to make sure everything stays in its place. We have a general rule that if things start to get a little untidy in wardrobes or drawers, take the items back out and check what the labels for those drawer dividers say. Make sure it's only items in that category that are being stored in that section. For instance, your underwear drawer gets used daily, and can get messy fairly quickly if you're not folding the items and putting them back into place correctly. So, if it does start to look chaotic, it's time to take it all out, categorise and put it away again. As hard as this might seem, don't let all the previous positive habits and organising go to waste. You can use the same steps you used in your initial detox, following The Process on pages 36–9. Instantly you will feel like a weight has been lifted – you have regained control and refreshed your memory of what you own and where it lives.

'SPRING' CLEAN

For some people, drawers and cupboards might start to get a bit unruly after a couple of months if they are high-traffic zones, like a toy room, kitchen utensil cupboard or sock drawer. But most of our clients benefit from a little freshen up of what we have originally organised for them about twice a year. Sometimes it works like a seasonal transition as the weather changes – people often like to have a spring clean to welcome the start of spring. The beginning of a new year is also popular when people seek to make a fresh start and put out the old to bring in the new.

However, a 'spring' clean doesn't have to happen in the spring and you can have one at any time throughout the year when you your instincts are telling you that a big detox and switch over is overdue. You may have left or switched your job, or your lifestyle or priorities have changed, and you no longer need a wardrobe full of work clothes, so it's a good time to have a clear out of unused stuff and work out whether you want to sell or donate any unwanted items. If you have a seasonal wardrobe, a good time of the year to bring in your spring/summer wardrobe is April/May and to then swap back to your autumn/winter wardrobe in September/October.

LITTLE AND OFTEN

Just spending a few minutes every day putting away items that have left their designated homes will make such a difference. If you let items get misplaced every day for a week, by the end of the week you'll have a lot more items to contend with and it can quickly become overwhelming, which can lead to your space getting out of sync. If you keep on top of any mess or clutter daily, or even tidy every other day, it won't be such a big job and you can get back to being clutter-free and organised quickly and calmly.

This is something that anyone can do when they have the structure in place, and it's so easy to follow. Working out where every item should live is like a big jigsaw puzzle that we help our clients to solve, and then it's down to them to keep the pieces all together! With a few folding techniques (see page 151) and an understanding of where everything goes, you can easily keep your home a calm and content space. The foolproof system you've put in place will last for years to come as simple techniques like labelling ensure that everyone knows where items live and should stay.

FINDING YOUR HOME STYLE

Interior design can sometimes feel daunting and the elaborate-sounding words can confuse you and make you wonder, 'What style am I?' It's important to know that there are no right or wrong choices – it's all personal preference. Deciding how to style your home can be tricky and there are so many styles to choose from that it can leave you not knowing where to start. The best advice we can give you is to always go with what you LOVE; it's all about turning your house into a home and small style tweaks can have an immense impact.

Finding your signature style may seem hard at first but it's all about being in tune with your tastes and not being distracted by what you think you should like. It's about what YOU love – listen to that inner voice that gives you an instinctive response when you look at a space and when you think about what you want it to do for your needs. This voice is what makes us all unique and make for an individual style – tapping into this will help you to create a space you can call your own.

The key to inspiration is for it to evoke an emotion. Start by thinking about what makes you feel happy and causes you to smile. Don't worry if it's not in fashion this season or on trend; it's all about finding what brings you joy and has a positive effect on your day.

CREATE A MOODBOARD

The first place to start is piecing together a vision moodboard of styles and items that you love, it's a perfect means for discovering your style in home interiors, clothes and fashion. Building a moodboard is a creative and fun way of collecting all of your ideas in one place and allows you to realise the styles and vibe you are attracted to and enjoy. Have an album on your phone, laptop or even a paper notebook where you can collate ideas, as inspiration can hit you at any point or anywhere. When you're out and about, watching a TV programme or reading a magazine, take note of what catches your eye. Pinterest is incredible for this as you can save a digital moodboard. The same goes for the save option on Instagram or you can look through interiors magazines and cut out items that inspire you. Once you have a collection of images, placing them together on a board reveals a clear overview of what you like. With this visual tool, you can quickly identify any common themes in what you have saved. This should give you a direction for how to move forward with your design or style tweaks as you can assess the colours, schemes and styles you have chosen and then think about you can introduce these in your home. This is the process we run through with our clients at the start of a project.

We like to start building our initial moodboards on Photoshop, where we collect inspiring images for the space and place them all together on a page to finesse an aesthetic to present to our client. Once this scheme has been agreed, we then get samples of the wallpapers, fabrics and paint palettes to produce a physical moodboard that can be held and touched. This enables the client to experience the textures and colours all working together and really helps to bring the new interior design to life.

INSPIRATION IS ALL AROUND YOU

When we start a design project, it always begins with finding inspiration and this can come from anywhere or anything. Take a little look in your wardrobe – fashion and interiors are closely connected. Whether it's packed with bold colours or monotone pieces, prints or plain items, when we look in our clients' wardrobes, we can quickly assess what style their homes will be just by the clothing hanging there. If your wardrobe is filled with colour and/or pattern, try to introduce this into your rooms in the form of wallpaper, textiles or even a brightly painted piece of furniture.

Take inspiration from places you love – it might be a restaurant, hotel or shop. Anywhere that boosts your mood and puts you at ease is a good place to start. Take photos of these places and add them to your moodboards. Think about what elements you like – is it the use of colour that lifts your spirit? The cosy textiles that feel welcoming and comforting? Are there features these places have in common?

top tip

Building moodboards is a brilliant starting point, especially if you are tackling a style vision room-by-room, as it will be less overwhelming but soon become obvious what the common threads are.

CHOOSING AND CONNECTING WITH COLOUR

Try to define what colours you love and those you instantly connect to – have a good think about how those colours make you feel on an emotional level.

Do you feel more connected to a neutral, natural colour palette or are you someone who loves bold and vibrant colour? A good way to establish this is by looking at your buying habits, flicking through magazines and creating a moodboard (see page 192) where you will be able to see if there are any common themes in colours you pick out. What shades have you been saving most?

Finding which colours you love does not always directly translate into using them all over your home, though. You may find you love orange, but you might not necessarily want orange walls as bold, bright colours can be overwhelming for a whole room. This is where accessorising comes in. You can weave in orange through artwork, cushions, throws or even with bolder pieces of furniture like a chest of drawers or sofa. The great thing about using colour in this way is that you can completely change the space as and when you wish without having to fully redecorate.

Using colour around the home is an expressive way to convey a mood, feeling, emotion or message across the various spaces and zones. We love using neutrals on walls because they are flexible and can be easily combined with lots of other colour pops and are adaptable for change if you so wish. They won't dominate, but will boost the sense of space and light.

Finding your style is not always permanent and your tastes can change over the years as you grow older and visit new places, not to mention the influence of new interior trends coming out every year. But as long as you choose items that make you happy and reflect your style, you will be able to keep your home in timeless shape. Your home should reflect you and your personality and be a place that you LOVE to spend time in!

WHICH INTERIORS STYLE IS RIGHT FOR YOU?

Below are descriptions of some of the most common interior style approaches. Have a read and think about which style you are drawn to – this will help you to formulate the right vision for your surroundings.

TRADITIONAL
Homey, symmetrical, timeless, calm, luxurious. Traditional design will often incorporate classic shapes from the past using older pieces of furniture like antiques or reproduction pieces. The furniture will be more ornate and fabrics heavier and more luxurious.

ECLECTIC
Quirky, fun, different, odd, varied. Eclectic style includes a mixture of lots of interior design styles over periods of time: different textures, colours, styles and trends. Interesting key pieces in the room add interest.

MODERN
Clean, crisp, sleek, simple and largely clutter-free. Modern interiors are simple in every element, using contemporary materials such as metal, glass and steel. Think minimalism with clean lines in your furniture choices yet make sure they are still comfy and inviting.

SHABBY CHIC
Vintage, distressed, feminine, nostalgic. This is a soft and dreamy style which embraces a blend of furniture and accessories that have a French twist with feminine florals thrown in with pastel neutral colours.

GLAMOROUS
Luxurious, textured, glitzy, sophisticated. Glam interior design is a mix of deluxe fabrics, classy metallics and a touch of sparkle! Accents of gold and glass and deep rich colours are a key feature of glamourous style. Think Hollywood and movie star vibes!

SCANDINAVIAN
Simple, minimalist, functional, textured, soft. Light muted colours with clean lines and simplicity, includes the use of natural materials such as wood and leather. No carpets but floorboards covered with oversized textured rugs is a common feature in Scandi living. Lighting is key; maximise the light in the room and decorated with cosy textiles.

The Style Sisters
Guide to styling your . . .

bookshelves

Bookshelves can be great not only for books but can house other beautiful objects and offer extra storage.

1. BOOKS
Books with attractive spines should be placed upright throughout the bookcase and you can even stack them on top of each other. It doesn't need to be overloaded with books unless you are trying to achieve a library look. Colour-coordinating your books and aligning and organising by size also looks cool and streamlined.

2. DECORATIVE OBJECTS
Adding vases, bowls and framed art is a simple way to add colour, personality and character. The shelves at eye level act as the anchor, so the most eye-catching pieces or loved items should be positioned there. Then work around those shelves mixing different height objects scattered across the shelves. Use items in odd numbers – the rule of three is important when it comes to interiors and styling (see page 200).

3. STORAGE
Decorative boxes are a brilliant way to get a little extra storage for smaller items that you don't want visible.

4. CUPBOARDS
Cupboards at the bottom of bookshelves are really useful for hiding away games, electronic appliances and any other items you don't necessarily want on show.

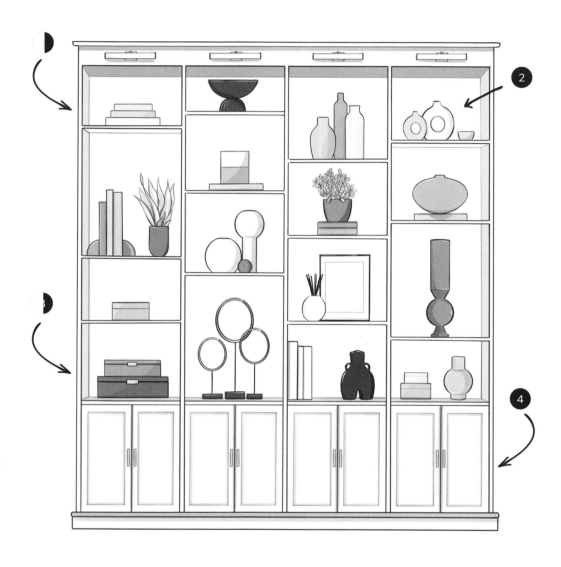

TOP TIPS for styling up your home

We spend a lot of time at home and it should be a sanctuary where you can refresh and recharge in a calm and cosy space that you have made your own. Our best advice is to fill your home with things YOU love – items that make you smile, textures you want to touch and scents that make you feel happy and uplifted. We want you to have a sensory experience every time you enter a room: we want your nose to be full of wonderful scents, your eyes to be drawn to colours, objects and textures, and even your ears to enjoy the sound of music.

In our designs we love to have a key statement piece that will give the room a wow factor. This could be an oversized mirror, beautiful bed, stunning pendant light or statement scatter cushions that add style. Below are some different aspects to consider that can help bring a bit of 'wow' to any room as well as helping to keep your home stylishly organised.

★ **LIGHTING IS EVERYTHING**
Consider the lighting in your home – statement lighting is one of the most important things to think about in a room and can transform the overall atmosphere. This can be done through the use of ceiling lights or lamps. Ceiling lights are a common and easy way to add light to a room, however downward light isn't that flattering on faces and creates lots of shadows. Think about placing spotlights on dimmers so you can set the tone at different times of day, and add wall lights, pendant lights and lamps for more of a feature and to create an ambience in the room.

★ **WHERE TO SPEND**
There are certain things in your home that are worth splurging on, for instance flooring and window treatments, whether it's blinds, curtains or shutters. They are key staple pieces for your home, which will stand the test of time. Flooring is a long-term investment, so opt for a colour that will work well with your planned scheme and that will suit other colours in case you redecorate in a few years. If you prefer carpet, go for the highest quality you can afford and choose one that feels great

beneath your feet and has a stain guard applied – think comfort and luxury as well as practicality!

★ **A TOUCH OF TEXTURE**

Bring touches of texture to a room with beautiful rich velvets, sheepskin throws or linens. These can add instant visual lifts even if the colours are all similar and the room is quite neutral.

★ **COMFY CUSHIONS**

For cushions, go for feather pillow inserts that are slightly larger than the covers as this makes the pillows stay plumper and gives you the perfect cushion to karate chop!

★ **GO LARGE ON YOUR RUG**

Always go for a larger rug as it will make the room look bigger. Smaller rugs in the middle of the room end up looking like a lost floating island.

★ **ADD ART**

Never underestimate what putting some art up on the walls can do. This is an inexpensive option; you can even get creative and frame beautiful pieces of wallpaper or fabric. This is an affordable solution to add colour to any room.

★ **MIRROR MAGIC**

Use oversized mirrors for instant light and glam. Mirrors used in small spaces help to bounce light around and the reflections will make it feel more spacious. We love to use a decorative mirror over fireplaces or floor-to-ceiling mirrors in hallways and dressing rooms to allow clients to check their outfits before leaving the house.

★ **PLANT POWER**

Bring life and colour into a room with plants and flowers. You can do this through faux or real versions depending on how green-fingered you are! If flowers are not your thing, consider dried flowers or pampas grass or palm leaves, which look great in tall vases.

★ **FLOATING FURNITURE**

Floating furniture away from the walls will actually make any room feel more spacious, this goes for shelving too - make the most of those walls.

★ **MAP YOUR MOVEMENT ROUTES**
All rooms should have a defined traffic flow. This is the path people will take when walking through the room and getting to different parts. It should be clear and easy to manoeuvre around without tripping over wires, seating and clutter! Avoid those blockages!

★ **CLEVER STORAGE**
Don't be afraid to think outside the box when it comes to trying to include more storage in the home. Consider decorative pieces of furniture for example. You could add a freestanding linen cupboard or a small decorative wardrobe. You can add shelves and paint the piece to suit the room it's going to live in, resulting in a beautiful, interesting piece of furniture that also gives you plenty of storage.

★ **ROUND TABLES FOR SMALL SPACES**
Round tables in small rooms make the space flow better and you won't bang your hips or legs on any nasty corners!

★ **ACCESSORISE**
Accessories are key when styling a space. Our go-to pieces when styling a room are coffee table books, vases, decorative boxes, candles, diffusers and ornaments. These look especially striking on a coffee table or bookcase.

★ **THE POWER OF THREE**
When styling a side table, bookcase (see page 194) or coffee table (see page 72), group items in threes and place at varying heights. You could place a candle, ornament and plant on a coffee table book, for example.

★ **CONCEAL YOUR CONTROLS**
Hide ugly thermostats, security systems and other wall-mounted controllers with a box frame on hinges so it's disguised as a photo frame but inside is the unit.

The Style Sisters
guide to styling your . . .

gallery wall

If the thought of adding a gallery wall to your home seems expensive or complicated, we're here to show you otherwise. The whole idea is for you to be able to display and hang beautiful prints, pieces of art or photos on your walls to bring life, personality and happiness into your home.

How you wish to display your chosen pieces is entirely up to you – you can have the frames all the same size, colour and style and displayed in a neat arrangement if you're into clean lines and symmetry or if you're going for an eclectic-style, you can afford to have a few different frames to add to the desired aesthetic.

Poster and art prints are an accessible way to inject colour and style into a room. There are lots of websites offering numerous prints that would suit every style out there, and what is great about poster prints is that you can update them easily and inexpensively if you fancy a change. There are also many amazing options of abstract images, sketches, photographic and themed prints available, so you're guaranteed to be able to find something that suits your taste.

If your frames don't come with a photo/picture mount, there are websites that can make mounts for your frames to the exact sizes that you need. We love the look of a big mount in a frame with a smaller image framed in the middle.

Some top tips before you get overexcited and start drilling or hammering holes in the wall:

1. Trace around your frames on to wrapping paper or kraft paper, then cut these out and you will have templates for your frames.

2. Place the templates on the wall using masking tape and curate your gallery wall arrangement – use the larger frames first as the anchor towards the middle, then start to place the smaller frames around the middle (see page 204).

3. Take a step back and look at your templates on the wall. Does your arrangement work well with the space? Is your eye drawn to a certain area? Do you need to break the images up a little more? Lots of smaller sized frames can look cluttered if grouped together, so make sure that they are evenly distributed around the gallery wall area.

If you feel confident and don't want to do the prep work with the templates, go with your gut instincts and use your creative eye to arrange the frames in the order and arrangement that you like. Just make sure you use a spirit level to check the frame is straight – they even have this an an app on your phone now, so it couldn't be easier to access.

An alternative to a gallery wall is a picture shelf. Attach a shelf to the wall and then position the frames on the shelf – you can use different sized frames and stack them in front of each other to create a layered look.

GOOD PLACES TO FIND STYLISH YET AFFORDABLE FRAMES:	FOR INTERESTING PRINTS THAT ARE ALSO GOOD VALUE FOR MONEY:
• **H&M Home** hm.com • **IKEA** ikea.com • **Zara Home** zarahome.com	• **Desenio** desenio.co.uk • **Fy!** iamfy.co • **Juniqe** juniqe.co.uk

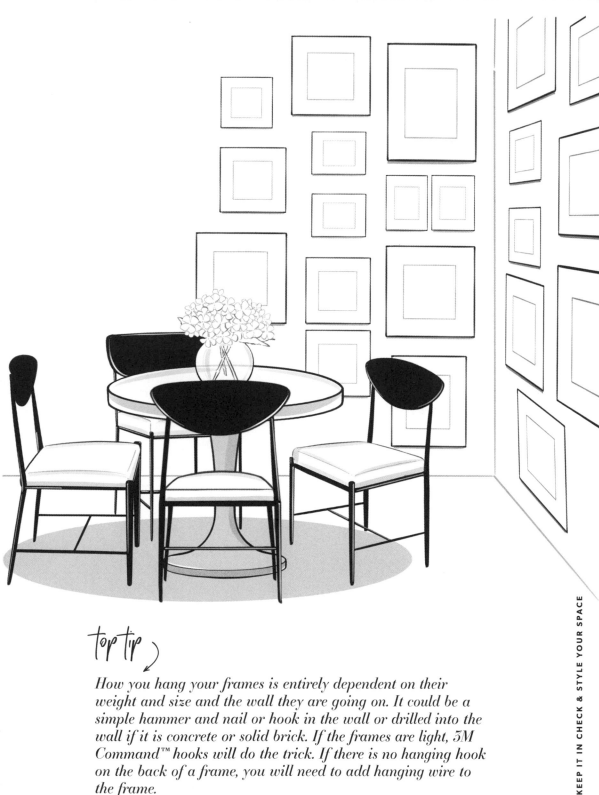

top tip

How you hang your frames is entirely dependent on their weight and size and the wall they are going on. It could be a simple hammer and nail or hook in the wall or drilled into the wall if it is concrete or solid brick. If the frames are light, 3M Command™ hooks will do the trick. If there is no hanging hook on the back of a frame, you will need to add hanging wire to the frame.

Our visual guidelines

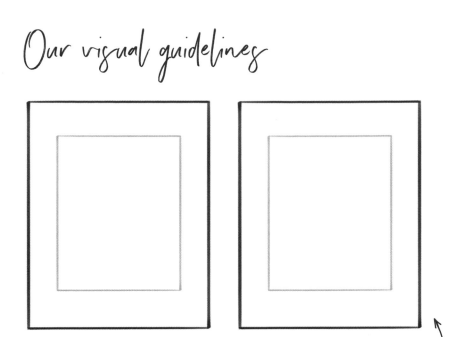

Leave a gap of 5–10cm (2–4in) between each frame as you want there to be an even gap between each frame

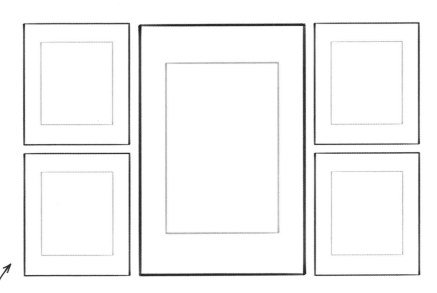

Artwork should appear as part of the overall design of the room and not seem to be floating so far above your furniture that the whole space feels disconnected

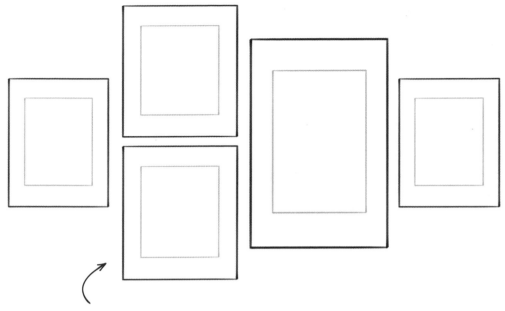

Make sure they are all straight and in line using a measuring tape and spirit level

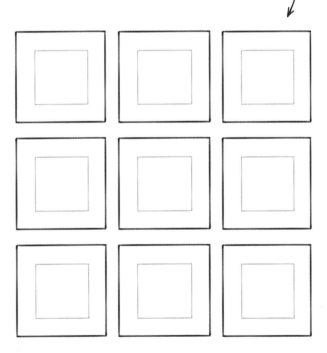

top ten

HOUSEPLANT IDEAS

Plants are such a simple solution for adding interest, texture and colour to a room and bringing more of the outside in, which is proven to improve your well-being – small wins with huge impact! These are our favourites:

1 Kentia palm

A great air-purifying showstopper plant to make a statement in a corner. Works best in rooms that get a lot of light, although not harsh sun.

2 Corn plants (Dracaena)

Works well in most light conditions apart from direct sun. Low maintenance as doesn't require much watering but enjoys humidity so particularly good for bathrooms.

3 Snake plant

An excellent all-rounder as works well in most light conditions and requires little water. Brilliant for bedrooms as it stores up oxygen during the day and then releases it all at night.

4 Peace lily

Works well in most light conditions, though will flower more in brighter spots. Loves humidity so a good bathroom option, provided it's not too dark.

5 Philodendron

Thrives in moist atmosphere so again a good choice for a bathroom and is fine in semi-shade.

6 Zamioculcas

Great option for darker rooms as doesn't require much light. Also, the less light it gets, the less water it needs, so the ideal choice if you're looking for a plant that doesn't need much care or attention.

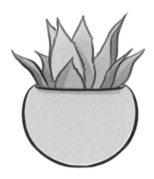
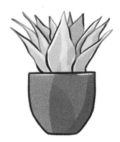

7 Parlour palm (Chamaedorea)
Easy to look after and do well in moderate to bright light, just not direct sun, so keep away from windows.

8 Devil's ivy
Good for darker rooms as it will do well in almost any light conditions, although it will grow quicker in a bright space. Another moisture lover, so a great choice for a shady spot in a bathroom or kitchen or on a shelf.

9 Fiddle-leaf fig
You can get small specimens to sit on tables or larger floorplants to make a real impact. It likes indirect sun, so perfect placed away from a window in a bright room.

10 Succulents
There are so many options to choose from, including architectural-shaped cacti. These are great for pretty much every room, from small specimens for your desk, to a pop of green on your bedside table or living room bookcase. A little collection of three also works well in any space.

BEST PLACES TO GET PLANTS:

★ **IKEA**
ikea.com

★ **Patch**
patchplants.com

★ **Leaf Envy**
leafenvy.co.uk

★ **Pointless Plants**
pointlessplants.com

FRAGRANCE FOR THE HOME

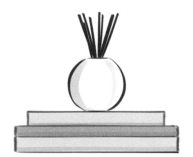

We tell everyone who will listen that fragrance is one of the most important aspects of your home. Scent is closely linked to our memories and our emotions and these can really influence what scents you choose for your home.

There are multiple options for adding fragrance around the home – candles, diffusers, room sprays, wax melts and wardrobe scents. Not only do they look amazing and add decorative touches to a room, but they also introduce a sensory experience to your surroundings.

Candles are a lovely decorative detail to fill your home with an aroma that you love. Candles can bring light to a room in the evening and add ambience to the space. Make sure the wick is trimmed and the wax burns evenly, and don't leave a candle in front of a draught or open window or door. If you have small children, then candles are a bit of a no-no, unless they are placed high up safely out of their reach. Do consider room sprays and diffusers which are a little more child-friendly. Again, it's best to store and display these out of reach of little hands if you can.

Candles vary in price and quality; the cheaper the candle the more toxic it can be, and some can even leave a black smoke stain on the ceiling. Opt for a natural wax like a soy candle if you prefer to use organic and/or natural products. Certain scents can be overpowering, smell intense and may give you a headache. If you can, try to invest in top-quality candles and perhaps only light them for special occasions to make them last longer. Don't forget you can reuse the candle jars once they are finished as a decorative ornaments.

Scent is closely linked to our memories and our emotions and has the power to really lift our mood!

Consider placing candles in areas you wouldn't necessarily think to put them (and not lighting them), like a linen cupboard for instance. The fabrics will absorb the candle scent and every time you open the door you will be welcomed with a lovely fragrance.

Diffusers are statement items and release fragrance all day long. If the scent is too strong, remove a few of the reed sticks and the smell will become less intense. Remember to turn the reeds every few weeks to stop them drying up.

Mist diffusers with scented oils are another genius way to add fragrance to your home. These can look lovely placed on a console table (make sure there is a plug socket nearby) and their fragrance will fill the air and create a beautiful atmosphere.

We like to use a variety of scents in different rooms around the home for different times of the day – this gives scented signals that direct you from work to leisure and day to night. Certain scents can be a real pick-me-up throughout the day and emit wafts of calm, concentration and cosiness into every corner of your home, from waking and using towels that smell clean and fresh in the morning to the relaxing spray mist on your pillow at night.

TOP TEN SCENTS FOR THE HOME

★ Jasmine
★ Lavender
★ Oud
★ Rose oud
★ Orange blossom

★ Lime & basil
★ Amber & ginger
★ Clean cotton
★ Green herbal tea
★ Bais berries

STYLE SISTERS

upcycling

When restyling your newly organised
space, you don't always have to look to
change a piece of furniture altogether;
sometimes it just needs updating.

It can be super easy to give something
a new lease of life and we are going
to share some of our favourite
ideas and hacks.

★   Upcycling is both sustainable and saves money, whether updating a piece of existing furniture or sourcing pieces of second-hand furniture inexpensively and then giving them a little TLC to bring them back to life, ready to be a part of a beautiful home again.

★   Older pieces of furniture like chests of drawers are often very well made and can also have unique details like engraved patterns, interesting shapes and unusual handles. Giving them a lick of paint can make them feel brand-new and can work out better than buying new. Depending on the style of the piece and the look of your home, don't be afraid to explore different paint types, such as chalk paint, or even just sanding the item down and oiling it.

★   We have used découpage to update pieces of furniture, which is such a clever way to create a statement piece. We recently used découpage on a chest of drawers from the 1970s using a modern geometric wallpaper. By doing this and then swapping the handles we gave it a completely new look. Check out the transformation on page 149.

★   Simply replacing the handles and door knobs allows you to update a piece of furniture instantly. We purchase handles from local DIY stores, online or from Etsy for more bespoke and unique pieces. If you're on a budget this is a thrifty hack to turn a cheaper piece of furniture into something that looks expensive.

★   Spray paint is another of our favourite ways to update furniture. We love a can of spray paint; we're always giving something a little spray so it fits in with the interior theme of the room we're styling. If you can't find a piece in the exact colour you want, consider giving it a few coats of spray paint for a perfect colour match. This is especially fun with smaller items such as vases – you can often find some cool older pieces in charity shops and then simply spray them so that they fit in with your colour palette!

GOODBYE &
GOOD LUCK!

Now you've detoxed your home and you're no longer holding onto the things that were weighing you down, your home should be feeling so much more organised and everything will have a clear place and home. You have styled your rooms and mastered our tools, tips and tricks... it's finally time to enjoy your new space! However big or small, your home should be your haven where you love spending time. You deserve to feel amazing and reap the rewards of the Style Sisters process – you've invested time, effort and maybe even money, so it's time to live your best life and, most importantly, enjoy!

Your home is an environment to refresh, recharge and relax. When things look and feel in control, you'll approach each day positively, with a clear head and a can-do attitude. This year has been so crazy and intense – achieving tiny tasks in the home and celebrating these wins is essential. We hope our advice brings you calm, comfort and joy amidst the chaos!

We want to thank every single one of you who has purchased and read this book from the bottom of our hearts. It's been a wild three years and this journey that Style Sisters has taken us on has been unbelievable – we are so thankful for every opportunity we've been given. We honestly believe that every one of you can add a little bit of stylish organisation to your lives. We've seen first-hand how detoxing and curating a clutter-free space can change people's lives and transform their mental outlook – and we hope that everything we've shared in this book helps you too. Even if you just use one or two tips, that makes us happy – spread the word, share the organisational love and don't forget the motto 'Style Sisters made me do it!'.

Lots of love

Gemma & Charlotte

x   x

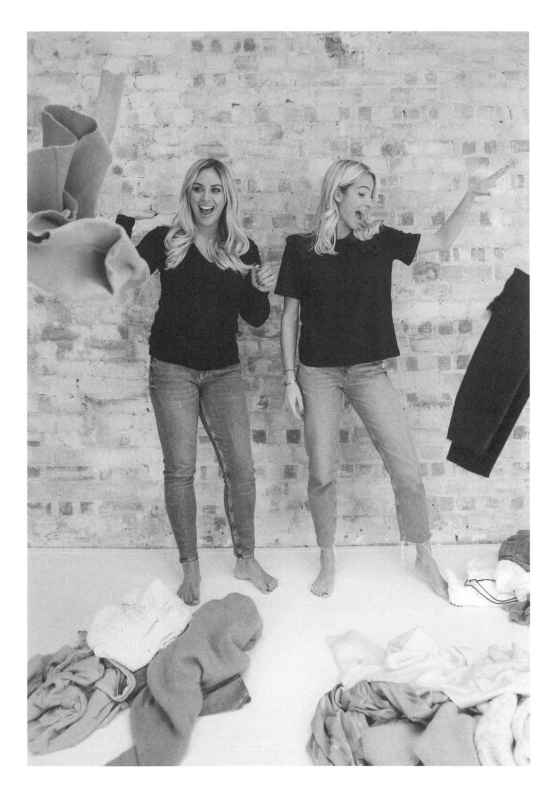

About us FAQS

1 **Are you actually sisters?**
Gemma – Sadly no, but we may as well be!
Charlotte – We are sisters in style.

2 **Which celebrity's wardrobe have you enjoyed detoxing the most?**
C – Ahh, we can't choose! If we're being honest, we have enjoyed everyone's. We know it sounds boring and cheesy, but we love what we do, and everyone so far has been really nice.
G – We love it when friendships are made while we're doing what we do. We've lost count of the number of times we've had wine and giggles with our clients – it definitely makes our job that much more enjoyable!

3 **Do you just do wardrobes?**
G – We detox, organise and style the whole home, often upcycling pieces of furniture. We love to make a space the best it can be.
C – We love to make over rooms. It's great when we not only get to organise the home, but do the interior design too!

4 **What is the strangest thing you have ever found at the back of a client's wardrobe?**
C – Ha, ha, ha, that would be telling!
G – We've seen it all though… It actually doesn't faze us in the slightest, everyone's human. We are always highly confidential, respectful and discreet.

5
Which celebrity's wardrobe would you love to get your hands on?

G & C – Anna Wintour's!

C – Could you imagine the cool stories she would have to share?

G – Not to mention the clothes!

6
What is your favourite room to design and organise?

G & C – The wardrobe!

C – We love to design beautiful dressing rooms and arrange the clothes like they are in a boutique.

7
Where do you get your inspiration from?

C – We take inspiration from pretty much anything; it could be a piece of furniture, a cushion or even a piece of art.

G – Magazines, Pinterest and even people in the street could all spark an idea. We are always taking notes and constantly observing.

8
Are your styles the same? How do you differ? How have your styles changed over time?

G – We are basically the same person! We both have very similar tastes. Our styles are definitely constantly evolving as we are always surrounded by lots of lovely different looks, however I will always love a neutral palette with pops of colour.

C – Same as Gem! My style has definitely matured over the years and since having kids we are both a lot more practical when it comes to interior design – storage is a must!

9
What's more important – style or fashion? How do you view both of them?

G – I don't think either one is more important than the other. Style is a way to express yourself – there are no rights or wrongs. Some of the most stylish people I know don't follow fashion or trends.

C – Style comes so naturally to some people, whereas fashion can be followed and mimicked. Being able to express yourself stylishly and timelessly is a true gift, yet fashion and style are so closely entwined.

10
Where do you see yourselves in five years?

C – Happy, healthy and still doing what we love. Style Sisters will be bigger and better – we will be selling products and helping lots more people!

G – I definitely see the business growing and growing and offering more services. We always planned for Style Sisters to be a lifestyle brand and for it to feature more services and products. We both love what we do so much and want to help and inspire as many people as we can.

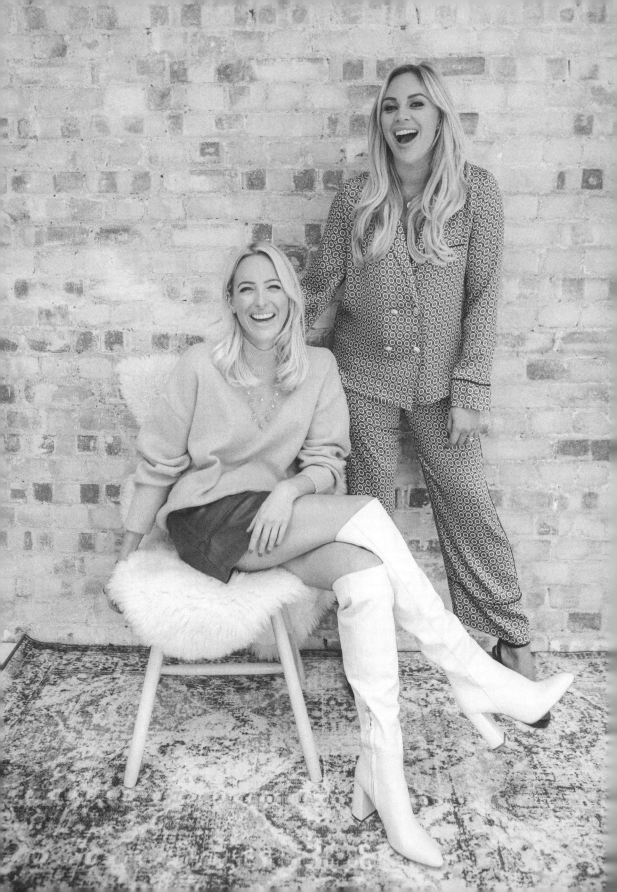

THANK YOUS

We are so incredibly grateful to each and every person that has not only bought this book, but followed and supported our Style Sisters journey so far, we just want to say a huge THANK YOU!

We never dreamed three years ago we would be lucky enough to be doing something we love every day, with each other.

The opportunities that have come our way from simply doing our passion is something we will forever be grateful for.

Thank you to every single person who has helped to make this book, we are so proud of it and couldn't have done it without the help of all those involved.

Thank you to our manager Lauren, who looks after us and whose main focus is making sure things align with our vision, we're so grateful to you for all you do for us and feel so lucky to have someone on our team who has the same beliefs and ethics as us.

To our families, we are so blessed to have each and every one of you! We are so thankful for all your love and unconditional support. Without you we wouldn't be able to do what we do. You are a huge piece to this puzzle.

Presley, Charlie and Hudson, we are so proud of you, thank you for being so understanding when us mummies have to work long days, everything we do, we do for you, we love you all so much!

Craig and Tony, thanks for holding down the fort whilst we work and for always supporting us on our Style Sisters journey, we would be lost without you!

Lastly, a huge thank you to our very special mummas. The list of everything you have done and do for us is endless and we are so grateful for you. We wouldn't be the girls we are today if it wasn't for you. We love you!

THANK YOU, from the bottom of our hearts for reading this book, we are two very happy and extremely grateful girls.

Lots of love
xx

OUR FAVOURITE PLACES TO SHOP

We're always asked about our little black book of shopping secrets and where we go to discover our best storage and interior finds. So, here's our ultimate list of our favourite places for online and in-store shopping, and where to get our Style Sisters must-haves! Enjoy!

AMARA HOME
A beautiful website with gorgeous home items – we could buy it all!
www.amara.com

AMAZON
If you need something in a rush, Amazon can be sure to save the day. It's our number one shop for our label machine, label tape and slimline hangers!
www.amazon.co.uk

ANTHROPOLOGIE
Cute and stylish items for your home.
www.anthropologie.com

ARGOS
Perfect place to click and collect items you need for around the home.
www.argos.co.uk

BELIANI
Amazing key pieces.
www.beliani.co.uk

BHS
They are still online with a classic collection of lighting.
www.bhs.com

COLDHARBOUR LIGHTS
The prettiest lights we have ever seen and beautifully hand made.
www.coldharbourlights.com

CULT FURNITURE
Cool, sleek designs for pieces around the home.
www.cultfurniture.com

DESENIO
We love buying stylish prints for our own homes and our clients from here. They do lots of stylish studio collabs!
www.desenio.co.uk

DUNELM
Everything you need for your home under one roof. We purchase our vacuum-pack bags here.
www.dunelm.com

DUSK
Beautiful bedding.
www.dusk.com

DWELL
Modern and stylish pieces for the home.
www.dwell.co.uk

EBAY

We have sometimes sourced sold-out products for clients from eBay from sellers selling new. It's always worth a browse and it's a great way to find cool pieces that people no longer want, perfect for upcycling!
www.ebay.com

ETSY

Homemade, beautiful and unique pieces for your home.
www.etsy.com

GREAT LITTLE TRADING CO.

Cute storage for kids.
www.gltc.co.uk

H&M HOME

We're obsessed with H&M's home range and every client of ours has at least one piece of H&M magic in their home!
www.hm.com

HABITAT

The place to find cool furniture and accessories.
www.habitat.co.uk

HEAL'S

The lighting and sofas are unreal!
www.heals.com

HOMEBASE

A great place to pick up anything DIY.
www.homebase.co.uk

HOMESENSE

You can only shop in store and every time you go you will find some interior treasures. Be sure to purchase there and then as items go out of stock very quickly.
www.homesense.com

iDESIGN

We would literally be lost without our iDesign products! We use them every day for an organised life – practical yet stylish. (Also available from Amazon.)
www.idesignlivesimply.com

IKEA

Our one-stop shop for photo frames and SKUBB drawer dividers!
www.ikea.com

iLITE LIGHTING

For gorgeous lighting.
www.ilite.co.uk

JOHN LEWIS

They stock a lot of well-known interior brands and you get a great guarantee on the products you purchase.
www.johnlewis.com

LA REDOUTE

We love the style of the home items and the rugs are lovely too.
www.laredoute.co.uk

LUXDECO

We wish we could buy it all!
www.luxdeco.com

MADE

We love the modern and clean designs.
www.made.com

MAISONS DU MONDE

Furniture and accessories for the whole home.
www.maisonsdumonde.com

MARKS & SPENCER

Classic style.
www.marksandspencer.com

MATALAN
They have a cool lighting section and home accessories.
www.matalan.co.uk

NEXT HOME
Cute pieces for the home.
www.next.co.uk

NOT ON THE HIGH STREET
We love purchasing from independent retailers collected on here.
www.notonthehighstreet.com

OLIVER BONAS
A selection of cool home items.
www.oliverbonas.com

OLIVIA'S
Beautiful items that we could browse and shop for hours.
www.olivias.com

RITUALS
The products are just the best – we love to put diffusers and candles in our clients' homes.
www.rituals.com

ROCKETT ST GEORGE
Cool, just cool.
www.rockettstgeorge.co.uk

SHABBY STORE
Lovely pieces for the home.
www.shabbystore.co.uk

SHROPSHIRE DESIGN
Lots of beautiful home items in one online store.
www.shrops-design.co.uk

SOHO HOME
Pure class; we don't need to say any more.
www.sohohome.com

STACKERS
Beautiful storage for the home.
www.stackers.com

SWEETPEA & WILLOW
This website is just stunning – the beds and sofas are unreal!
www.sweetpeaandwillow.com

THE RANGE
Anything you need for around the home you can find in this shop.
www.therange.co.uk

THE WHITE COMPANY
Bed linen, furniture and photo frames are our top picks from here.
www.thewhitecompany.com

TROUVA
A selection of lovely home items from independent shops selling online.
www.trouva.com

WEST ELM
We love to source decorative pieces from here.
www.westelm.co.uk

WILKO
Shop online or in store for storage baskets and other organising items.
www.wilko.com

WORDERY
A top place for us to purchase coffee table books.
www.wordery.com

ZARA HOME
Effortlessly cool and contemporary pieces.
www.zarahome.com

First published in Great Britain in 2021 by Yellow Kite
An imprint of Hodder & Stoughton
An Hachette UK company

1

A CIP catalogue record for this title is available from the British Library

Hardback ISBN 978 1 529 34725 8
eBook ISBN 978 1 529 34726 5

Editorial Director: Lauren Whelan
Project Editor: Isabel Gonzalez-Prendergast
Copyeditor: Vicky Orchard
Designer: Nikki Dupin at Studio Nic & Lou
Illustrator: Sally Faye

Printed and bound in Italy by L.E.G.O Spa

Hodder & Stoughton policy is to use papers that are natural, renewable and recyclable products
and made from wood grown in sustainable forests. The logging and manufacturing processes a
re expected to conform to the environmental regulations of the country of origin.

Yellow Kite
Hodder & Stoughton Ltd
Carmelite House
50 Victoria Embankment
London
EC4Y 0DZ

www.yellowkitebooks.co.uk
www.hodder.co.uk

Goodbye from us and big love!

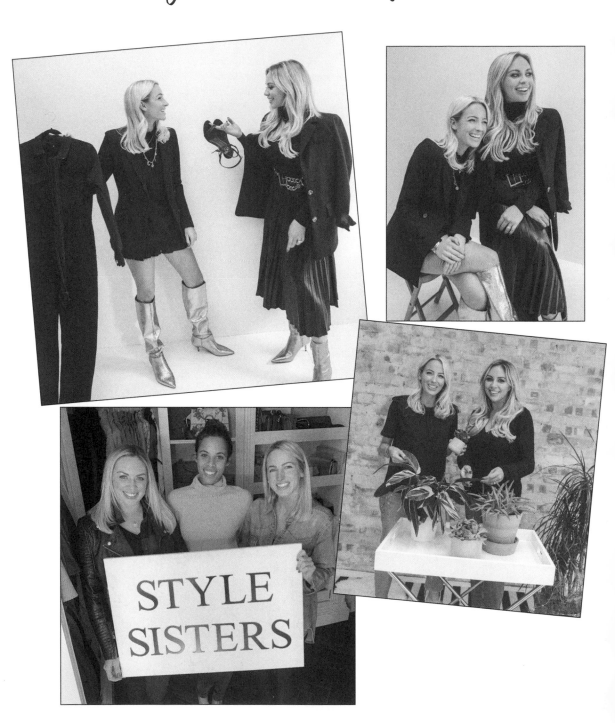

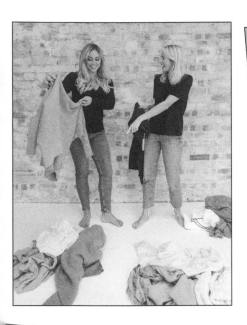

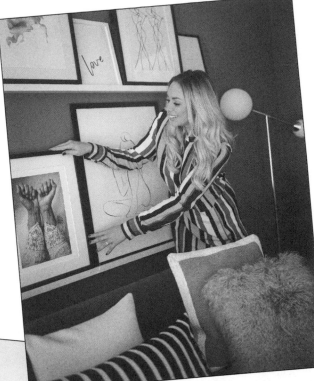

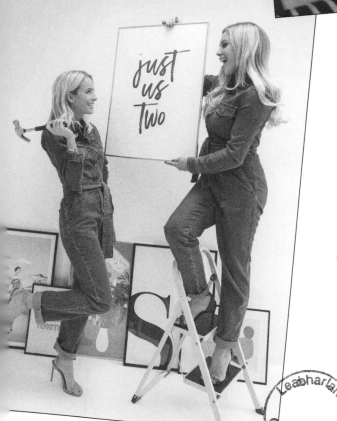

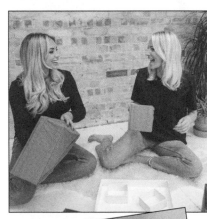

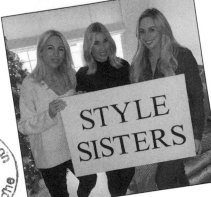

just us TWO

STYLE SISTERS

Leabharlann
Contae na Mídhe

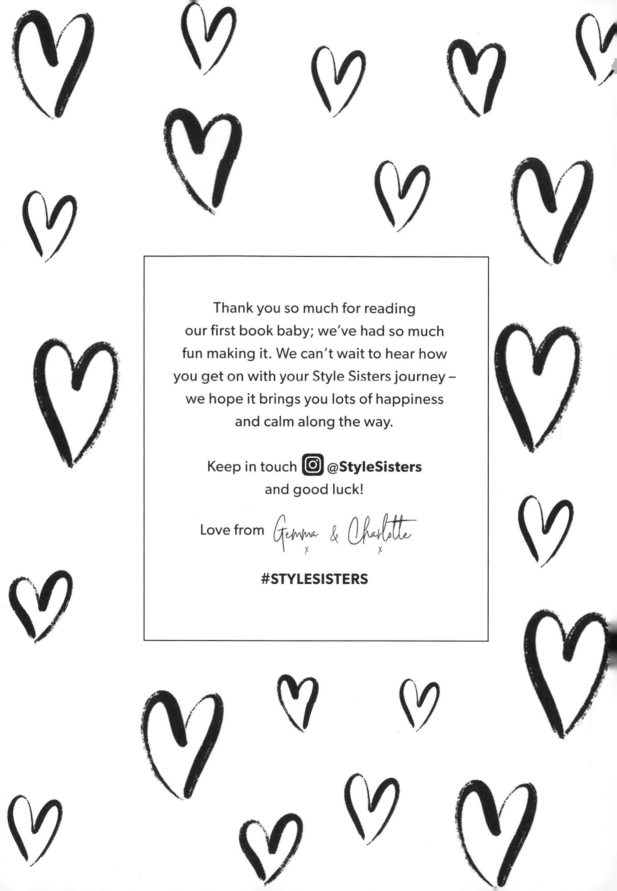

Thank you so much for reading
our first book baby; we've had so much
fun making it. We can't wait to hear how
you get on with your Style Sisters journey –
we hope it brings you lots of happiness
and calm along the way.

Keep in touch 📷 **@StyleSisters**
and good luck!

Love from *Gemma* & *Charlotte*
              x   x

#STYLESISTERS